Nine Months to Go

What You Need to Know

Dr. Joann Richichi

Oakley Publishing Company, Inc.

Copyright © 2009, Joann Richichi

All rights reserved. No part of this book may be used or reproduced in any manner whatsoever without the written permission of the Publisher.

Printed in the United States of America.

For information address:

Oakley Publishing, Inc.
140 Broadway, 46th Floor
New York, NY 10005

Library of Congress Cataloging-in-Publication Data

Richichi, Joann

Nine Months to Go/Joann Richichi

Library of Congress Control Number: 2009921704

p. cm.

ISBN: 978-0-9818400-3-1

First Edition

10 9 8 7 6 5 4 3 2 1

Visit our Web site at
http://www.oakleypublishingcompany.com

Praise for *Nine Months to Go: What You Need to Know*

Dr. Richichi's illuminating and entertaining book on pregnancy care contains a wealth of information that women who are expecting or may conceive in the future will find useful. It is filled with easy to read straight talk from an experienced OB/GYN who very effectively weaves in her great sense of humor with a perspective that can only be gained from many years in practice. Many complex medical topics are presented in a readable manner with an abundance of practical advice based on current standards of obstetric care. This book is a must read for all those yearning to know what to expect during pregnancy, especially those who appreciate a lighthearted but technically accurate and often humorous approach to the topic.

—Joseph N. Bottalico, D.O., F.A.C.O.G. (Dist.)

This book provides pertinent information about pregnancy and delivery and yet manages to be the funniest medical text that I've ever read. As Dr. Richichi's colleague, I can attest to the fact that she has mastered the art of establishing the doctor-patient relationship. She does it again in *Nine Months to Go*. As a mother and a physician, Dr. Richichi skillfully, and with humor, balances science and real life experience, making this a must read for every pregnant woman. The honest, ask-my-friend-the-doctor approach gives additional reassurance and accurate interpretation of facts. Other physicians can complement their practice with a book that is lighthearted and will make readers laugh as the journey towards life's miracle unfolds.

—Juliet M. Nevins, M.D., M.P.A., F.A.C.O.G.

Dr. Richichi has brought a book that is head and shoulders above the rest. It should be subtitled "A Girlfriend's Guide to Obstetrics…and My Girlfriend is an Obstetrician and Mother!" There are numerous confusing aspects of pregnancy that she brings a common-sense approach to in an easily read format. For my money, the part that stands out ahead of the pack is how she effectively describes the confusing area of prenatal screening and diagnosis for genetic abnormalities and makes it understandable.

—Ronald J. Librizzi, D.O.,
Chief, Maternal Fetal Medicine, Antenatal Testing Unit,
Virtua Health System, Voorhees, NJ

This book is lovingly dedicated to my first son, **Alexander Anthony Chianese**, for allowing me to experience both the burdens of pregnancy and delivery as well as the rewards and riches that follow. Thanks to him I did all this a second time and was blessed with **Nicholas**. I love you both.

Acknowledgements

There are so many people who have helped contribute to the successful publication of this book. You all know who you are, but I would like to give special thanks to my children for putting up with me while I had the occasional computer glitch and subsequent fit that required their assistance and patience "right away." Especially poor Nick, who unlike his brother, didn't have the luxury of being away at college when I needed help. They also didn't seem to mind the many take-out dinners during the writing and re-writing of this book. They are so special to take pride in their overworked mother's eccentricities and accomplishments.

I would like to thank my office manager and friend, Marie Hernandez, who knows how to deal with me better than anyone I know. She knew when I needed her to drop everything so I could get things done with "the book." She was a pleasure to have in my corner even though I was a bear to have in hers.

I would like to thank my business partner and best friend in this world, Dr Marianne DiGiovanni (Mare), for her support and for reading what to her was Obstetrics 101, over and over again. Her unfailing belief in me helped push me in the direction that I needed to go to confidently finish this book. I would like to thank my wonderful office staff for their never-ending input, support and dedication.

I sincerely would like to thank my publisher, John Lewis, for seeing the life this little book was meant to have, and for believing in it and in me. He truly made my dream a reality. I would like also to thank the rest of the team at Oakley, especially Jennifer Adkins and Eric Lindsey for their willingness to change things over and over again at my request.

I would like to thank my sixth grade teacher and longtime friend, Stephanie Andrus, for helping me believe in myself and giving me the courage to follow my dreams.

Thanks to my parents, Helen and John Richichi, who always had faith in me and helped me succeed in being who and where I am today. I love you.

I must thank Sandra Harkins. She typed the very first draft of this book from my dictation before I got so proficient at typing. She not only encouraged me to move forward on this endeavor, but she also taught me how to experience the joys of the Internet.

Most of all I would like to thank all my patients, who shared so much of themselves with me throughout the years. If not for them I would not have had the foresight of things that need to be known, nor the hindsight to see the humor in this wondrous aspect of life. I am sure so many of them will read between the lines and know that they came to my mind as I found the words to express their deepest fears, silliest questions and most neurotic concerns to all of you. Thank you all.

Contents

Foreword……………………………………………….. ix

Why I Wrote This Book……………………………………...xiii

Chapter 1: *Great Expectations*……………………………………1

Chapter 2: *To Be or Not to Be*…………………………….. 21

Chapter 3: *I've Got You Babe*……………………………….50

Chapter 4: *It Happened One Night*……………………...........87

Chapter 5: *Happy Days Are Here Again*……………….…... 101

Chapter 6: *She's a Brick House*...125

Chapter 7: *No Way Out*...155

Chapter 8: *A Hard Day's Night*..165

Chapter 9: *Blue Moon*...183

Foreword

If you are pregnant or just thinking about it, I would like to share with you my knowledge and my experience, as both an obstetrician and a mother. I'd like to also offer you reassurance in this exciting, beautiful time filled with a multitude of emotions and anxieties. I have been very frustrated in my years of practice with patients who use various books as bibles. What I'd like to tell them is what I tell my residents in training: medicine is not black and white. There is a lot of gray. There may be five paths to take to the same solution, all of which might be very different but have similar outcomes. Every patient is unique, as is every circumstance.

The Internet oftentimes is a wonderful source of information, but it can also be a hindrance to both patients and physicians alike. We all know that there are web sites and chat rooms for just about anything. Answers to a variety of questions could be at your fingertips in seconds. So than, why read the book? Why listen to the advice of your practitioner?

The answers are simple. A lot of the information on the Internet is not always accurate, and it all may be way too much info to digest and assimilate. I am by no means trying to insult your intelligence. It is just that without medical training, you may misinterpret the answers to your questions. Many of you who are reading this book are not health care professionals. Relax and leave all the details to the practitioner whom you have chosen to have faith in.

I am not a lawyer. I couldn't possibly imagine reading the wealth of material that a lawyer would have to have read in his or her years of training to know the answers to so many legal scenarios. And in truth, I wouldn't want to waste my time trying to know. To me that stuff is boring and just plain hard to comprehend. If I sit down to read something legal, I find myself thinking about the shopping I have to do, or even the laundry I hate to do. I would even rather cook then read that stuff. I know I would have a poor interpretation of all that, which to me is mumbo jumbo. I would never imagine being my own lawyer. Not only do I have an extreme lack of interest in legal matters, but I find it all way too anxiety provoking. I would always rely on the expertise of those who are well trained in dealing with legal matters. I encourage you to do the same with your pregnancy.

Try your best to keep away from the chat rooms, because they are a broader extension of the old wives' tales that are still circulating among many families throughout the world. So in an attempt to prevent you from experiencing the anxiety of information overload, my goal is to be minimally scientific and mostly sensitive about delivering to you the informative you need to know. I hope I am able to reach the emotional and psychological needs of the expectant parents who read this book.

The purpose of the book is to make you aware of what is normal and alert you to the things that you should make your practitioner aware of. I hope to do this in a very accurate yet condensed fashion.

The important thing is never to panic, because this can be a wondrous time for you, full of anticipation and optimism and some stretch marks, hemorrhoids and varicose veins—but, oh well, they're worth it! Unless you are planning on birthing more than ten babies, pregnancy will encompass a very short time in your life, so please try to enjoy it.

Keep in mind that throughout this time it is important to maintain an open line of communication with your obstetrician or nurse midwife. We will talk more about that in Chapter One. This is a personal time for you and your significant other. You must feel comfortable with the practitioner you choose. That person should never make you feel as though he or she is insensitive to your questions or your needs. Let's face it—if you don't feel comfortable, you are going to turn to the Internet, and then you will really be screwed. The Internet just doesn't cut it in the warm and fuzzy department. I have never thought it a source of comfort.

NINE MONTHS TO GO

Remember, you may have to ask many questions to relieve some of your overwhelming concerns. As I tell my residents, obstetrics is a five-year residency; obviously there is a lot to know. Therefore, it shouldn't be your job to know everything there is to know simply because you're pregnant, but rather, to feel at ease with what will eventually occur.

Most of all, remember to enjoy it, for goodness' sakes. Details and facts are not important, as you are not a student. I don't care how intelligent you are, if you are a rocket scientist or have an IQ of 160! You must remember now at this point in your life you are an emotional, intelligent, frightened and insecure wreck of a woman.

Facts are not going to describe what it feels like if your doctor tells you that you need to deliver early because the fluid around the baby is diminishing, or that you need an amniocentesis because your sequential screen (which we'll talk about further) is abnormal. Therefore, it is my hope to combine my knowledge as a physician, my emotions and concerns as a twice-expectant mom, and the fears of a knowledgeable hypochondriac (that would be me), all in one easy-to-read, simplified yet comprehensive book. This unique combination is here now for the first time ever so that I can make YOU better aware of what to KNOW while you are waiting to deliver so much joy into your life.

Remember when you are reading this book that I was there and I know it can be frustrating, especially if you don't do it like the book says. Very few women do. They don't usually gain the 22-28 pounds that we recommend. They tend not to exercise because they're too tired, have swollen legs that look like tree trunks and hemorrhoids which get oh so much worse when squatting. They don't eat fish or take omega-3 fatty acids or fish oils because, after all, the supplements are too big to swallow, and who the heck wants to burp fish all day long when you're fighting the gas problem that has suddenly built to the point of extinguishing the small city in which you reside? They're never in labor for just five hours, nor do they push for just ten minutes.

Joann Richichi

If you are fortunate enough to be able to follow all the recommendations and suggestions made by your practitioner and have an uneventful, easy pregnancy and delivery, Great! More power to you! Then perhaps you've wasted time, money and energy reading this book! But I do hope you got some laughs along the way.

Remember, this book is aimed at helping you through those times when you just can't bear down anymore from chronic constipation. And those times when you are at a birthday party and bend over to pick up the birthday present as you pass wind in the birthday boy's little face, who just happens to be sitting next to your child, whom you have now embarrassed for the rest of his life. It's aimed at helping you come to terms with the fact that you are now fat and flatulent! Its goal is to help you deal with the times that you went to speak with your girlfriend's husband and burped up the tuna hoagie you had eaten several hours before.

As you read this book you will come to realize that my pregnancies were really not a fun time for me. And as we go through this book together, I'll elucidate for you all the many reasons why I wasn't a happy, smiling pregnant lady. That doesn't mean, however, that pregnancy can't be fun for you. It does mean that I understand where you are coming from when you are just too fatigued to enjoy the anticipation of your little precious gift. My hope is that if you read the words from a mother and a doctor, you will be informed and comforted through what I consider hell for forty weeks.

Oh, and by the way, if you have already done a pregnancy successfully, and a friend has you read this foreword, and you think that pregnancy was the most fun, fabulous and enjoyable time of your life and that you would love to do it over and over again no matter what complications arise, God bless you! This book is of absolutely no value to you. But if you are somehow given a copy, give it away to your not so fortunate girlfriends.

...Enjoy!

Why I Wrote This Book

If you read the foreword, you now have an idea as to why I wrote this book. But by way of further introduction, I'd like you to know a little about myself. I have two teenage sons, Alex, age 19, and Nicholas, age 16. When they were little I was an extremely busy obstetrician in a two-person group. Back then my demanding schedule put me on call every other night and every other weekend. All that my kids ever wanted was a "real mommy," the kind that stays home, cooks and cleans. Somehow, despite their wish having never come true, these two wonderful guys still love their mother. Remember that for me to have been given this enriching opportunity of having special guys to love in my life, I too had to undergo the humbling experience of being pregnant and giving birth.

I am now fortunate to be in a four-women practice group, which affords me the additional time to explore some of my eccentricities and hobbies, one of which is writing. I was motivated to write this particular book from having written several articles for our obstetrical-gynecology journals. Most of my colleagues found them interesting and informative. Patients and friends who read them liked my writing style and found it easy to read and enlightening. What I liked about writing them was that I enjoyed being able to reach people and send a message. *Nine Months to Go* was given birth to as a result of my overwhelming desire to reach as many people as I possibly could.

My practice is still very busy, and I love what I do. I also am fortunate enough to have great business partners and to now be on call every fourth or fifth night. That for me is a true luxury that affords me the opportunity to write. The combination of my lighter work schedule and the fact that my older, very needy son is now away at college affords me the luxury of having the free time I never thought I could possibly achieve.

Joann Richichi

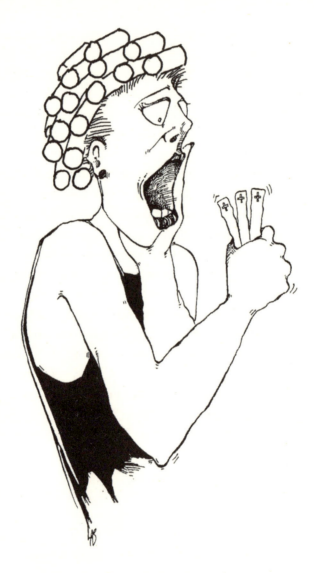

I guess this means I'm pregnant?

NINE MONTHS TO GO

I sincerely disliked being pregnant, probably because I had just about every pregnancy-related complication known to women. I am also very impatient: I couldn't imagine waiting nine months for anything, let alone getting my energetic, not-so-slim body back. The experience was, however, obviously worth it.

To a certain degree, I feel I could have done it better if I had only done it one more time. However, my ex-husband was not willing to again undergo the agony I caused him while I was pregnant. No matter what, I couldn't convince him that the third time I could get it right (one of the many reasons why he is now my ex). Instead, here I am deciding to put my years of training and experience to a very fruitful cause, and that is to let *you know what you need to know* about this very exceptional time in your life.

As a physician who loves her work, I can truly say that I am blessed by the opportunity to have so much fun bringing life into the world each and every day. I feel that I have been truly gifted to have this opportunity. This short, fleeting time in your life should also be fun for you. But, instead of my witnessing the enjoyment in many an expectant couple, I have been disheartened on many occasions by the patient who has been confused and made anxious by reading various sections in the multitude of books that have been written on pregnancy and related issues. While I know it was the intention of these writers to inform the public, the scientific fashion in which they did so tended to allow for worry and speculation.

The Internet, although a source of great information, can also be a source of unneeded anxiety caused by the outpouring of informational overload. Let's face it: there is a lot of stuff out there, and sometimes it is hard to weed through what is actually important and necessary to know. It is my job here in this book to elucidate that information for you and to dispense with the trivia that breeds confusion.

In addition to the anxiety-producing Internet and literature, the family friend or old Aunt Sally can make your life and mine quite miserable by relaying some old family wives' tale that is just downright absurd. These tales are sometimes so believable that it takes me a lot of time to reassure the patients and set them back on the right track. This book is an attempt to put things into perspective by combining the simple viewpoint of a woman who has been there and didn't like it with the knowledge and experience of a doctor. I will try my best to diminish your concerns by making you aware only of *what you need to know*.

It is obvious that patients nowadays are much more inquisitive than they were years ago. The general public is more educated, and they want to learn what to expect. No one wants to be kept in the dark as they were in the past. The philosophy back when my mom was pregnant was, "What you don't know won't hurt you." My grandmother would tell me she didn't want to go to the doctor because she was afraid they would "find something wrong."

My grandmother delivered six of her eight babies at home, and when she was 42 she had a set of twins delivered by an old midwife with a dirty, blood-splattered apron. While she pushed in the back room of her small Brooklyn home, she was happily oblivious to the things that could potentially go wrong. She didn't worry about the fact that she was at home without the availability of anesthesia or that an operating room was ten miles away. And she didn't have a clue how the mode of delivery could possibly affect the IQ of her breech twin, and she didn't care.

That is not to say she didn't care about her children—she most certainly did. Life was just a lot simpler then, and people didn't tend to be so competitive. Most people didn't go to college, and if they did it wasn't remotely difficult to get into a good school. Now if your kid's SAT scores aren't 22,000 or better, you can kiss not only Ivy League but your top college choice bye-bye. To be a woman who went to college would make you unique, to say the least.

My grandmother was not concerned about the possibility of hemorrhaging and needing a blood transfusion. Birthing babies was just a part of life, and you wouldn't be a typical stoic Italian wife and mother if you didn't do it without moaning and complaining. Back when I was a resident in obstetrics and learning about all the things that could potentially happen at the time of childbirth, I was amazed by her courage, or perhaps her simplicity and blind faith, all of which enabled her to deliver at home.

My curiosity led me to inquire more about the details of her births. I asked my Nan and my great aunt, who was there at the time of each birth, about the circumstances of her deliveries. They both made them all seem like such a piece of cake. The irony of it all was that things could have happened back then that could have been potentially devastating. And yet, so many of us and our parents are walking around without devastating handicaps from our not-so-monitored births.

Just as an example, with the birth of my grandmother's twins, the first one delivered breech and the second one was head down. In this day and age we would never allow such a combination to deliver vaginally. This particular scenario could be problematic, because the two chins could become locked with one another and, therefore, both babies would not be able to descend into the birth canal. Fetal distress could occur, or failure to progress, both of which would necessitate a C-section, which would be hard to accomplish in a small back bedroom of a Brooklyn home. While in the hospital setting, this potential complication could be quite easily handled, at home it could have been fatal to all involved. Until this day I am still amazed that all my aunts and uncles have relatively normal to above-average intelligence.

In the course of her storytelling, I was told of the profuse amount of bleeding that my grandmother had endured after her deliveries. When I asked what they did for her while she lay at home bleeding, my aunt answered that they gave her a "shot of scotch." That was just what she needed to dehydrate her more, but it was a good remedy to help dilate her constricted blood vessels. When I told my grandmother that I was going into the field of obstetrics and gynecology, she asked what I'd be doing. When I explained that I'd be doing surgery and delivering babies, she looked at me and said,

"Do they really need doctors for that stuff nowadays, Jo?" And here I was thinking I would be saving the world.

Of course I was interested in what was done in my field of practice "in the old days," so I asked my mom about her pregnancies. She told me that with her second pregnancy (my brother), she was reading in the doctor's office when her bag of water ruptured. My mother claims my brother's foot came out while she was in the waiting room and that the family doctor took her to the back of the office, where "he pressed on my belly and pulled out your brother."

My God, some of my residents have not even seen a breech birth because the risk of fetal injury is so high. And this was done in the office without a fetal monitor and by a family doctor who had limited experience in obstetrics. Today, the litigious climate in which we live would have a field day with that situation. So many things can go wrong with a breech delivery, and this story just baffles me. I was amazed at how far the field of obstetrics has come since my birth, and we won't say just how long ago that was.

When my mom spoke of her pregnancy with me, she said that I was very late—three weeks past her due date. We now never let a pregnancy go beyond two weeks past the due date. If we do allow someone to deliver after their due date, we do testing. The results of the fetal testing may or may not allow that pregnancy to progress further. Because my mother wouldn't go into labor on her own, a shot of Pitocin was given to her in the doctor's office, and she was sent home to labor. Again, totally unheard of these days because of the possibility of fetal distress and hypoxia (loss of oxygen to the brain). I often tell my mother that I might have been a genius had she not been given that shot.

So while the philosophy of "what you don't know won't hurt you"—and believe it or not, oftentimes it doesn't—is still the philosophy that some of the older patients like to abide by, the pregnant population now is in a never-ending quest for knowledge. They love to be taught. Therefore, because I like to teach, I made an attempt to do so with this book.

NINE MONTHS TO GO

However, when I told my friends and family that I was taking on such a time-consuming project, they all knew they were in for trouble! Once I have it in my head to do something, that's it—it's done. I get a little consumed by my projects, or as my kids would say, obsessed. I tried my best not to sacrifice time with anyone that I care about, and I tried to show them throughout this book how much their help, guidance and support meant to me. I can only say that I hope I have succeeded.

So to those of you who decide to read this book, I hope you find it as interesting, light, funny, reassuring and informative as I intend it to be. I certainly do hope that you are in no way offended by its content.

Also, let me say that I don't know about you, but when writing I get very tired of saying "him/her." Therefore, when I refer to physicians, I'd like to generalize by saying "he" so that I can't be accused of being a chauvinist. Hope that's okay with you.

Joann Richichi

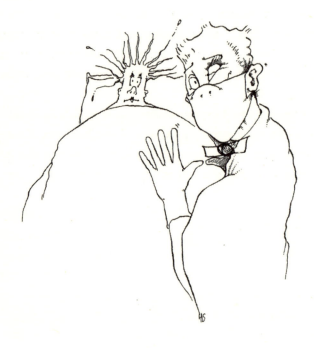

Hello... I am Dr. Bernie Bush. So happy to be at your cervix, I mean service.

Chapter 1

Great Expectations

Choosing Your Physician

Choosing your obstetrician is not as difficult a task as choosing your partner. Looks, height, personal interests, cultural background, ethnicity and eye color really are of no value or importance. Thank goodness, or I'd be in trouble—especially when it comes to the height. However, personality, sense of humor, warmth, understanding, compassion and level of intelligence should be weighted seriously. So then, how do you distinguish which caregiver is right for you? Before you decide, there are several issues that should be of extreme significance to you:

1) Of what kind of practice do you want to be a patient?

2) What qualities would you like your doctor to possess?

3) What type of patient are you?

4) Is your doctor Board Certified or Board Eligible?

5) Who referred you to that particular doctor?

6) What hospital(s) does he practice out of?

7) Is the doctor well known in your community?

8) Do you want a doctor or a nurse midwife to deliver your baby?

It is important to speak with friends and relatives who enjoyed their particular obstetrical experience. Some of the best physician referrals come from patients who have been to and liked a particular doctor's style or bedside manner and who felt comfortable with that doctor. Perhaps the hospital he practices out of is too far from home or you don't like what you have heard about the hospital. If you truly like the physician, it can't hurt to take a tour of the facility to become more familiar with what is available and what to expect. If you trust in your caregiver, the facility may not be as big of an issue. Many hospitals are redoing their obstetric wards in a constant competition to make the patient rooms as homey and comfortable as medically possible. (Lucky you).

If you are comfortable with the practice you choose, then you will know that they will be delivering you at a location they feel confident with. The unit you deliver at may not have all the amenities or allure of some of the birthing centers you have read about, such as a Jacuzzi tub or flat screen TV. But it will have the practitioner and a staff who will take care of your needs as well as your baby's.

Some patients choose the facility over the physician. Some patients are lucky enough to have both of these important aspects to their liking. If you chose the facility as a starting point, you can ask for recommendations afterwards. That is a more than viable option, especially if you are new to an area and have heard great things from other people who have delivered in a center near you.

I am a D.O. (doctor of osteopathy), and so is one of my partners, Marianne DiGiovanni, with whom I have practiced for 21 years. We have two additional partners, one of whom is an M.D. (medical doctor), the other a D.O. The difference in title has never posed an issue at our office; however, it is not uncommon for a patient to ask about the difference between a D.O. and an M.D. In theory, subtle differences may exist, but in actuality we are the same. We do the same surgical and medical rotations; we have the same internship and residency programs. Most hospitals have a complement of both types of physicians.

NINE MONTHS TO GO

The difference lies in the philosophy behind the osteopathic practitioner. The teaching incorporates alternative medicine and a more natural approach to the healing arts, i.e. vitamin therapy, spinal/muscle manipulation, and relaxation. We follow the same guidelines and do the same surgeries as our M.D. associates. Many D.O.'s, however, do not abide by the osteopathic philosophy because it is not always a practical approach to modern day, patient-oriented problems.

I believe in the benefits of western medicine. However, because illness has, in my mind, always been caused by a multitude of factors, I tend to try to incorporate these osteopathic principles into my practice whenever possible. Our body parts are all connected. Somatic illness can have many origins. Manipulation of the musculoskeletal system and the spine can help decrease and even eliminate some of the culprits of illness.

To elucidate the components of this theory, I will use a medical condition most of us have heard about: PMS (premenstrual syndrome). There are advertisements out there that talk about the various medications that can help control this disorder, thereby preventing your partner and family from wanting to extinguish you for your horrible behavior. These commercials are so good and graphic that after I yelled at my kids for not helping around the house (certainly a justified reason for any mom to take a fit), my son told me, "Mom, maybe if you took that stuff they talk about on TV, you wouldn't get so angry and upset," and my other son agreed. "Yeah, Mom, maybe you should take it. It's just one small pill a day." Jeez, just who's the gynecologist here anyway?

While I believe in the effectiveness of medication, I often try to start patients on a more natural regime, like vitamin B6, evening primrose capsules, vitamin E, and exercise with diet control and weight loss. Often, patients are not willing to do what is necessary to take the time to make themselves feel better. They want a quick fix. That attitude, coupled with the growing pharmaceutical industry, often makes holistic approaches to treatment fall by the wayside. The teaching and practice of this medical art is, however, quite useful and can be very rewarding for the patient.

If credentials are important to you, I am sure you will be able to acquire a lot of knowledge about your physician on the Internet. Keep in mind when you do your search that nothing beats word of mouth. While someone may look very appealing on paper, it is important to know how he communicates with and treats his patients.

Recently I had to have carpal tunnel surgery. Although I had felt the worsening symptoms of my ever-narrowing tunnels for quite some time, I put off surgery for as long as I could because I was truly afraid. I was worried that my nerve would get accidently cut, and if that happened I would no longer be able to do surgery, write, or paint. I would have to give up all the things I loved most. These fears were for the most part irrational, and although the physician in me knew that, the patient in me was a basket case. This surgery is relatively common, and usually accomplished with very few complications. However, I thought of myself as a surgeon who was in need of the best of the best, because after all, my hands were my life!

So I went to the best of the best. He graduated from Harvard medical school and practiced in Philadelphia. He was written up all over the Internet as being a world-renowned hand surgeon. His office was plushly decorated. Before I even met with the doctor, his assistant looked over my medical records and said, "Well, obviously you are in need of surgery. The doctor's schedule is quite booked, but he can do your surgery in two months." I looked at her like she had two heads and thought, *No way am I going to wait two months*. I was so numb I couldn't even hold a toothbrush, let alone a scalpel.

When the doctor introduced himself to me, he never made eye contact. In the course of the interview, he was very abrupt, and he had a matter-of-fact attitude towards me and the cutting of my gifted hands. When I asked him if I would be able to adequately perform surgeries once my own surgery was done (on both my precious little hands), he looked at me and said, "Young lady, do you know who you are talking to? I am world-renowned, and I have operated on over 300 surgeons."

What an arrogant SOB, I thought. With that I said, "Do you know who you're talking to?" and I got up, picked my coat up off the chair and left without a moment's hesitation. Well, actually I did have one tiny hesitation, but that was only because he said I was a "young" lady...

After that unrewarding and nerve-wracking experience, I talked to a few nurses at various surgery centers in the area. As I asked around, the same name came up several times. This office was also in Philadelphia. The difference was that this doctor came out to the waiting room. He had the sweetest, kindest eyes, and he held my numb, tiny hand in between his big, warm, paw-like hands and said, "Don't worry, I know you are nervous, but I will take good care of you. We doctors tend to be worrywarts when it comes to ourselves. We can do this as soon as you would like. Believe it or not, I can get you right back to work in no time at all."

In less than one minute I was ready to go under the knife, because I knew this man was going to help me. Yes, maybe I am a big baby, but this guy knew that however minor this surgery was to him, it was a great big deal for me. He cared. And he was a teddy bear, but that was what I needed. In my own office I have a lot of my awards and diplomas displayed on my wall for patients to see if they so choose, and he did as well. I realized after I left his office that I had never even glanced at them, because you know what? I didn't need to.

So keep my little story in mind when choosing your physician. As you can see, it is also important to know what type of patient you are. Had I realized I was a wimp, I wouldn't have wasted my time with going to see the arrogant SOB I would have asked around for the caring teddy bear. Most of us don't always know what we need, but hopefully, this chapter will help you figure this out. When thinking about the type of physician or practitioner you may hope for, you may want to consider these questions:

1) Would you like a father figure?

2) Would you like that person to respect your decisions in pregnancy management and in the labor process?

3) Do you feel intimidated when you ask that particular doctor or practitioner a question? Or does he make you feel comfortable and at ease?

One of my partners and I have worked together for many years now. We practice very much alike. Our belief systems are similar, as are our ethics. We believe in a physician/patient partnership. We don't like to do anything unless it needs to be done. For example, we never use forceps unless there is a risk of fetal compromise. We both firmly believe in pain management and that a patient should enjoy the experience of labor, not have to endure it. We are both confident and extremely competent, and we have a busy obstetrical practice together while separately seeing a multitude of our own gynecological patients.

However, our personalities are extremely different. My partner tends to be much more direct, blunt and to the point. Her patients love her for her honesty, and they know she truly cares about them. I, on the other hand, tend to be more delicate in my approach to a patient's problems. I tend to tell the truth in a more "cushiony" way, and this tends to comfort my patients.

Some patients prefer the more direct approach. I once gave the results of a suspicious mammogram to a patient of Dr. DiGiovanni's while she was away. I told the patient my recommendations and what she needed to do next in order to have the proper follow-up and treatment plan. Of course, I tried to reassure her.

After I was finished going over the results with her, she was polite and thanked me, but she went on to say, "Dr. Richichi, you can make a malignant metastatic brain tumor sound like a walk in the park. I really would like Dr. D to call me when she gets back in town."

At first I was a little taken aback, but in time I realized (as hard as that might have been for me) that not every patient is going to like my style. And the differences are what make the world go around. That patient needed to hear it straight and to the point. That is why it is important to choose the doctor who is right for you. Our other two partners are a complement of both of us. The combination works for our patients and seems to help us to all get along.

When you have four women together, all with strong personalities, watch out. There always has to be an alpha dog, but that is definitely not me. Yet we are fortunate to work very well together. We respect each other's opinions and always put the patient first. One of us (and I won't say who) likes to get manicures, pedicures and massages. It seems she always has an appointment for one or the other. She says it relieves her stress. But no matter how stressed she may be, if we need her or a patient needs her, she will give those luxuries up in a heartbeat. Different personalities might attract very different patients—and we do. However, if one of my partner's patients gets me while in labor, the patient is very comfortable, and vice versa, because all of us have learned the art of medicine.

Now you may think the art of medicine is just dealing with medical problems and performing necessary surgery, but that is only part of it. The true art of medicine comes into play when a physician somehow understands the patient's needs and works with that patient. And although there are times when the patient's needs may prove to be draining and difficult to that particular physician's personality, the true artist is able to deal with that patient in a respectable, sympathetic, encouraging fashion. And believe me, that can prove to be a difficult task at times. However, if done from the heart, it will prove to be rewarding for all involved.

Unlike most relationships where we are told opposites attract, that doesn't seem to happen in the physician/patient relationship. In this case, "likes attract." There is a symbiosis that develops between physician and patient. The physician recognizes certain things in that patient that remind her of herself.

Now, I talked to you a little bit about the type of physician or nurse midwife you should choose, so it might help you to see which category of patient you seem to fit into. Most physicians do not really categorize their patients. I have made up these categories as a result of my personal dealings and observations throughout my years of practice. They are meant only to help you and guide you on your quest to find your practitioner. Your physician will not categorize you when he makes rounds with his colleagues. He may, however, make note of your mental instabilities, issues, needs and concerns.

If you are a patient of mine, please do not get paranoid or insulted. Remember what I said about the symbiosis that exists wherein the physician sees similarities in that patient and vice versa. There is a mutual respect that oftentimes develops. Therefore, if I categorize you and you feel offended by this, remember I, too, am more than likely in that very same category! For example, there are:

1) The wimpy whiners

2) The loony-tunes

3) The laid-back, experienced types

4) The intellectual piranhas

5) The career-oriented neurotics

6) The perfect prisses

The wimpy whiners—They're mine! They cry, they complain, they are scared about everything, and they suck the blood right out of me! They tend to be very nervous. Remember that symbiosis I spoke of? The wimpy whiners are very often the leeches on the poor, innocent animal that happens to swim in the swampy waters, or they are the little birds that pick the bugs off the hippopotamus while taking a free ride. Nothing makes them happy. They always find something to complain about. Their head hurts, they have pressure, hemorrhoids, nosebleeds, swollen hands, swollen feet, swollen toes. They tell you about every ache, pain and bodily activity right down to the time and nature of the very last fart. But they are very appreciative when you help them and take the time to reassure them. And they have good, kind souls. (I have to have some justification for my actions.)

The loony-tunes are usually very happy, but irrational, hyperactive and emotional. And when they ask a question, you wonder if they have spent the last three years of their life on Mars. They are the ones who might ask if eating too much Jell-o can make the baby turn red. Or they might wonder if reading novels about homicidal killers could make their baby have those tendencies. Or better yet, if watching werewolf movies could make their babies hairy. Or my most favorite question of all time might be asked by these precious souls: "Could the baby see us while we are having sex?" If they don't like the answer, or if the physician is not thoughtful and sensitive to their very real concerns, they may have an unexpected and irrational outburst of tears, followed by a temporary fit of madness (they tend to be mine too—so I guess that tells you an awful lot about me).

In labor, I was very whiny. I complained, I was difficult, I didn't listen to anything that my physicians told me to do. I was a wimp who knew it all. The combination can be lethal. There was even a time when I dosed my own epidural just so I didn't have to feel the pain. I was thankful and quite happy to be helped, but I was also a nervous, emotional wreck. I questioned everything. When the doctor didn't deliver me at just the moment I felt I needed to be delivered, I had no problem clearly enunciating some of the most often used words in the English language.

Considering that I had to work with most of these people who were at the delivery, I embarrassed myself, to say the least. The cool, confident physician they were used to dealing with no longer existed; she was replaced by a 5-foot-2-inch, mean pregnant whale.

Even to this day, 19 years later, when one of my patients feels embarrassed about the way she is acting in labor, the nurses quite adamantly say, "You should have been here when your doctor was in labor!"

My pregnancies were complicated by preterm labor. I was given medication to stop labor at 31 weeks. I knew that this medication could affect other muscles in my body, making them weak. This is why we don't allow people to walk around when being given this drug. Their legs can be wobbly and buckle out from under them. Also, the medication can make you feel dizzy and disoriented.

Knowing all this, I insisted on getting out of bed to go to the bathroom. I was in no way going to move my bowels in a bed pan, in a hospital where everyone knew me. Needless to say, my legs were like Jell-o. I got out of bed anyway, because after four days of lying down my *arse* was so numb I couldn't feel it. Considering how big it was, I had an awful lot of numbness going on. I walked the halls like a crazy, pregnant drunk lady with an IV pole in one hand and a yellow purse (my Foley bag) in the other. I nearly fell, and would have had I not had a resident there to catch me and sit me down in a wheelchair like a good little girl.

This medication that I am speaking of is called magnesium sulfate, or "mag," as we docs like to refer to it. It is for the most part a good drug for its purpose. Having experienced this medication's darker side, I personally despise it. Therefore, I try to use it only when no other alternative is available. Although great at stopping the wrath of preterm labor, it can also slow down your gastrointestinal tract. I somehow thought I would be immune to all of this drug's potential shortcomings. After being in the hospital several days, I was hungry one night and decided to eat a pepperoni pizza with some resident friends of mine. I'm sorry to say that pizza was with me, my fellow residents and the labor/delivery nurses for a long, long time afterwards.

Needless to say, the **laid-back, experienced type** is what every doctor wants to get, but seldom does. Very few patients fit into this category. Their visits are short. They never hound their doctors and they rarely ask a question. They are sociable and happy to see you. Usually they have had at least two other children that delivered free of complications and at term. Those children are now running around the house and driving them crazy. They have very little time to worry about the nuances of this pregnancy.

As far as my partner's patients go, one gets the **intellectual piranhas**. You know, the type that reads everything and has been on the Internet a million times, yet knows nothing. This is the kind who tells you the way she wants things, and if it happens any other way, she might attack without the least bit of provocation. She knows the answer to everything and only asks a question so she can disagree with you. And she also has a date book or Blackberry and a ten-page birth plan that she carries with her everywhere. The birth plan has stars in the margins and is highlighted with either passion pink or brilliant yellow.

One of my other partners gets the **career-oriented neurotics**. They can almost be worse than the wimpy whiners and the loony-tunes because they are never really happy. They're always so worried about what life is going to be like now that they have this new addition. How will this impact their career? Did they make a mistake? What are they doing to their bodies? What are they doing to their minds? They can't think right anymore! They read everything there is to read, and they're scared about it all. They tend to be nice and they never disagree or argue with their physician. They really respect their doctors and take their advice, if for no other reason than fear of not doing so. The intellectual piranhas tend to blend with this category. Most of these patients tend to vacillate in and out of both categories simply because the wealth of knowledge can make the intellectuals very neurotic.

The sixth category is the **perfect priss**. They tend to be very good patients, the reason being that they listen to everything their physician tells them to do. They are the ones who tend to gain the appropriate amount of weight, who tend not to get bloated, who always seem to have relatively easy deliveries. They never bother their physician, and they hardly ever ask a question. They are together, or at least they want the doc to think that they are. They will never read this book. If they do happen to be given a copy, they will skim it and think it to be stupid (but that is okay, because I like them anyway). They also will have a perfectly-shaped belly, and they are the ones that everyone in the waiting room envies. As far as I'm concerned, we can never have enough of the perfect priss, since she does tend to make our lives easy and she does tend to have uncomplicated deliveries.

But all kidding aside, I can categorize patients simply because I've been there and because I've been a little bit of it all. I should consider myself lucky—I got to be every patient type in the book and got to experience every possible complication with just two pregnancies. Remember, pregnancy can be a nerve-wracking experience for most every first-time mom. Therefore, putting you in one of the patient categories I mentioned is not meant in any way to belittle you or make you feel insecure about the wide swings of emotions you are feeling daily. I respect them, and I respect you. That is why I can talk about all of this so honestly.

Now that you can see that you may fit into any of these categories, you can better realize the type of doctor or practitioner that might support and/or tolerate such behavior. The wimpy whiners and the loony-tunes want a "girlfriend" or a teddy bear. They tend to go with the midwife who is going to spend a lot of time and energy with them, or with a doctor like me—down to earth, comforting, reassuring, gentle, and one who will never yell at them. One who likes to listen, and who is generally shorter and more neurotic than they are.

The laid-back, experienced types can deal with just about anyone. They oftentimes prefer the gentle, confident, blunt physician like my partner. They don't need anyone beating around the bush —least of all their own. They want to hear it like it is—no fu-fus allowed! The intellectual types would in no way tolerate Marcus

Welby, M.D. The career-oriented neurotics tend to tolerate the father figure, but only if "Daddy" doesn't tell them what to do.

Remember, as many patient personalities as there are, there are that many doctor personalities to match them. Find the one you feel comfortable with. Comfort is a key issue. You don't want to be made to feel small or intimidated. (Well, maybe you might want to feel a little bit smaller.) You don't want to feel during the time of your delivery that your doctor doesn't care or doesn't want to be there. You want someone who understands your needs, and someone who respects your position—I mean that literally.

These are the issues that are most important in choosing your practitioner. Obviously, I used my own practice as an example since it is very familiar to me. I found it best to describe my experience in dealing with many different personalities. Keep in mind, however, that your choice may render you in a very different type of practice situation.

The next question is, do you want to utilize a group practice, or would you like to deal with one particular person? It depends on the group. If it has five members and you have been a gynecology patient of just one of the five, you might not like the fact that while pregnant you may have to rotate your visits between your doctor and his four other associates. Most practices do require that you do this so that you can be comfortable and familiar with your delivering physician. Most multi-member practices also have a rotating on-call schedule. Therefore, if you have not rotated your visits you may run into the awkward situation of having a physician you have never met delivering you.

If you don't like the idea of having to rotate, then you might want to choose a single practitioner. Keep in mind that this doctor will have to have some time off. You might want to find out who cross-covers him on those occasions. If you don't mind having to meet new doctors, and once you do, you happen to like the other four doctors in the five-person group and feel comfortable with them, then you should stay with that group. But if there are questions that you have regarding care, and if the doctor you really want will not be available for your delivery, than it is best that you seek a different group with perhaps fewer members.

If a doctor works solo, the questions you should ask him are:

1) Do you go away for weekends and/or do you have a life?

2) Do you cross-cover? And if so, with whom?

3) How many vacations per year do you take?

4) Are you planning on a vacation around the time I deliver?

Unlike being treated for other various medical problems, having a baby is a personal experience, and it is important to know and feel comfortable with the person who is delivering you. I can't emphasize this point enough.

The next question you should ask yourself is, would I like a midwife? If you would, most midwives are more than capable of handling normal deliveries under normal circumstances. However, anything that becomes difficult or high risk should go to the practitioner who covers that midwife. If circumstances become complicated, you might have to have the covering physician deliver your child. You don't have to meet the doctor. If you trust your midwife and have confidence in her, then you will also have confidence in the doctor she chooses to cover her. Also, the nurse midwife will almost always remain with you no matter what situations arise. Most of the midwives I have covered have been kind, caring, supportive and knowledgeable individuals. They make themselves totally available to their patients. While you are in labor, your midwife won't be bothered with ER calls or needing to attend a surgery. Her soul job will be you and your labor. You alone are the "Princess"— you and the five other people she may have in labor.

Before you make the decision, however, to go to a midwife, you should ask yourself if you are looking for a practitioner who is trained to handle every conceivable complication of labor and delivery. If you are, then the midwife, no matter how wonderful she may be, is not the one for you. If, on the other hand, you are looking for a more natural approach to the labor experience, perhaps having a midwife should be the route you chose. You should make sure she is licensed and certified and that she will be the one doing your delivery. Although all states license nurse midwives, some hospitals do not allow them to deliver. Believe me, in this day and age those hospitals are few and far between.

If you have had a prior C-section and wish to see a midwife, that is fine, but remember that the doctor may need to use forceps or vacuum on you, or you may need a repeat C-section. The current trend, which has been enhanced by the litigiousness climate in which we live, is to do a repeat C-section, unless the patient is adamant about an attempt at vaginal birth and meets the criteria to do so.

Some practices have midwives see the patients obstetrically in the office, but these particular midwives aren't the ones who will be doing the actual delivery because they are office-based midwives. Be sure that your group allows you to see the practitioner who will be doing your delivery.

You may be offered a nurse-practitioner during one of your office visits. The nurse-practitioner is office-based and will never perform a delivery. We have a nurse practitioner who was first a labor and delivery nurse. She worked at that capacity for 25 years before she went on for further training. She is quite capable of answering most if not all obstetrical questions and doing routine obstetrical visits. She does sometimes see our OB patients if she is not overwhelmed with her own GYN patients. The patients are given this option if we are running behind and they don't want to wait or can't wait the additional 15 minutes it might take to see one of the doctors. The patients love her. She is great. However, they are informed that she will NOT be delivering their baby. Knowing this, a patient may or may not opt to visit with her for a routine obstetrical visit.

If you are scared, you need someone who is understanding and reassuring. If you are a naturalist, you will probably like an open-minded physician who believes in alternative medicine and won't poo-poo your thoughts and wishes. You and your doctor must share some of the same expectations. If you feel more comfortable making a birthing plan and talking it over with your doctor, I would encourage you to do so. This experience should be based on a partnership. In order for it to be a happy and rewarding experience, you must be comfortable with your ability to communicate with the people whom you have chosen to care for you.

Another important issue that always seems to come up is, do I want a man or do I want a woman doctor? Sometimes my patients say, "I'm so glad I have a woman obstetrician to deliver my baby." Although I am happy that the patient may find comfort in my gender, I sometimes feel a little insulted by that assertion, to be perfectly honest. What should matter is that your physician is qualified and makes you feel comfortable, is experienced and knowledgeable, and cares about you and your baby. Their ability should not be based on gender. After all, I might get hairy in my old age. Then what? If I grow a mustache, will they still like me?

I do realize that some patients really want and get comfort from someone who has been there or has the potential to be there. They just want to know that you too have had a huge, cold, metal speculum pushed up your vajayjay just like them. If you choose on the basis of gender, however, don't lose sight of the other very important issues and qualities that I just mentioned. I hope you find the doc that will be your rock.

I truly value the opinions of my office staff, so I had them read Chapter One before I decided to go further with this endeavor. I suppose I wanted to hear, "Jo, we loved it—it was funny—I couldn't put it down—can't wait for you to write more—looking forward to seeing you on Oprah!" But instead there was complete silence. Having never written a book before and being sincerely excited to do so, I suppose I was slightly disturbed. "Okay, guys. What is it?" I asked them.

"Well, Jo, your patients are going to be mad, insulted, hurt and disappointed when they realize that they might be a loony-tune!"

Being open-minded and able to take a limited amount of criticism (even though it killed me), I asked what I should do. Should I be serious, boring, less graphic, more coy?

"YES!" was the overwhelming response. I sat and thought about it for some time, but didn't want to risk being mundane and, hence, less interesting.

Have you ever heard the expression, "You either love it or you hate it"? Whether it refers to an item or a person, that particular subject immediately becomes appealing to me. It oftentimes is multi-faceted and is, therefore, intriguing and exciting. That was my intention with this book. So I decided to leave Chapter One as is, and if you do choose to read this book, don't throw it away. Remember, the paper is recyclable and won't be a complete waste.

What you are now about to read is my attempt to rekindle your faith in my purpose and to put my very loyal and currently worried office staff at ease by categorizing the doctors, just as I have done to the patients, so you can better see to whom you may wish to open your heart, and then some.

Being a physician allows me the latitude to see my colleagues in a different light that may be somewhat iridescent at times. In my opinion, there are six doctor types; therefore, if luck is with you, you may find your perfect match. Remember, doctors, like patients, tend to be a blend.

1) Dr. Dapper Dan

2) The arrogant SOB (remember him?)

3) The jolly jester

4) The tough teddy (or maybe not so tough)

5) The studious stiff, a/k/a the nerd

6) The smooth sailor

I do believe these titles are somewhat self-explanatory. Numbers 1 and 2 I couldn't possibly get along with as a physician or as a patient. These are the doctors I now ignore, and they are the ones I butted heads with when I was a resident. The patients that tend to gravitate their way are usually the laid-back, experienced types, occasional loony-tunes, and a rare neurotic. Also, those looking for an authoritative figure may find themselves in the care of this type of physician. You can well imagine how an intellectual piranha or a career-oriented neurotic might clash with these stereotypes. The wimpy whiners just will not get the comfort and understanding they crave. On the other hand, the jolly jester and the tough teddy are usually warm and vibrant, less regimented and more flexible. The wimpy whiners just love these guys.

The tough teddy will keep the wall between you and him, but certainly will keep you secure and comfortable. If the tough teddy lets down his wall (as they often do), he may appear to be less professional because of his overwhelming warmth and concern. Just realize that he is a kind, caring person who only wants what is best for you.

The smooth sailor is so laid back, it is sickening. Remember, all the medical students are "Type AAA" personalities, so be careful of the smooth sailor because it is likely that he may at some point have had a nervous breakdown or may be on high doses of lithium. Occasionally, the intellectual piranha may gravitate that way because they can tell him what they want and oftentimes get it—anything goes. "Hakuna Matata"—don't worry and hang loose (so to speak). But can you imagine a neurotic in the hands of "Dr. Par Four—push if you feel like it"?

I know that about now you're wondering where I categorize myself. Sorry. I can't do that. It's up to you to decide.

There is one other physician type that I didn't categorize, and that is because there are so few of this type around these days. Managed care and the litigious climate have killed him. At one time all physicians could have categorized ourselves as the **compulsive-idealist**, but this category is slowly becoming extinct; therefore, I didn't list him as one of the commonly found physicians. If you are

NINE MONTHS TO GO

lucky enough to come in contact with one, you will recognize him because of his overwhelming concern, tender heart, lack of sleep and willingness to commit himself whole-heartedly to the care of his patients.

Now that I have equally insulted my patients and colleagues, let's go on to our next chapter, "To Be or Not to Be."

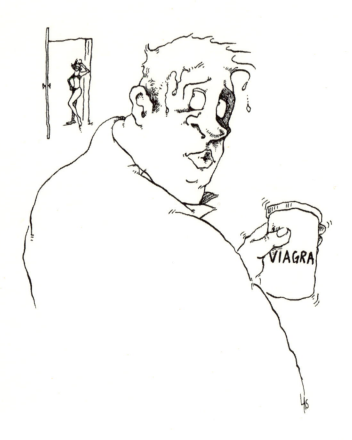

What happened to the good old days of romance and making love when we were in the mood? No wonder I have performance issues!

Chapter 2

To Be or Not to Be

OK, you're here! You have decided to give up your lifestyle of comfort. You too have fallen prey to the call of Mother Nature. To that inner desire to reproduce and replicate that which you liked well enough to now be able to control and improve. The magnitude of your desire to look into the eyes of God's creation and see through that mirror your own soul has overcome you. When you have that beloved creature in your arms at 3:00 a.m., and he pees on your chest and screams in your face, you will barely remember life as it was: peaceful, serene, devoid of anxiety, terror, humiliation and worry. When on the next day you awake and look at your bloodshot eyes encircled with the dark halo of sleepless nights, you will thank God for the miracle and pray that you will be able to survive.

Actually, some nights it may seem that bad, but having survived the infant days, I will say that the joys and happiness you will experience in your future as a result of your decision will be overwhelmingly rewarding. Therefore, eliminate any fears you might have of what you have done to your once-complacent life. It will only get better from here.

However, you just might want to eat your meals more slowly before you deliver. And you might want to take your time in a hot shower, because once you have your child, those seemingly mundane events will be a blessing to achieve. Don't want to scare you, just prepare you for the simple fact that pooping by yourself will no longer be an option.

Since I know you know *how* to make a baby, I will point out some important issues that you should consider prior to conception, as well as certain circumstances or medical and family history that you should make your practitioner aware of. Even though you may not be there yet, thinking is preparing, and preparing can be fun and limit your anxiety.

Things to think about BEFORE it is done

This chapter is designed to help the Type A person prepare for pregnancy. Some people prepare by knowing what to expect. Others treat it like they would getting an off-season golf course ready for spring. They feel the need to mow the lawn, pick the weeds, water the plants and feed them with all the healthy minerals to promote growth. And of course, we mustn't forget to cut the bushes.

However, if you want to prepare yourself, I know that for most of you, there are things you are wondering about and losing sleep over. The answers should be in this chapter and in later chapters as well. I also mention some things in this chapter that are common issues for most women to obsess over later on in their pregnancy. (If there is an element of repetition in the book, it is intentional. I repeat myself simply because you need me to say things over again.) When you finally become pregnant you will be preoccupied. Most of the time you will find it hard to focus on just about anything for longer than five minutes. So have no fear—we will try our best to make it all really clear.

More than likely, if you are reading this you have either decided to conceive or you are newly pregnant. If you are pregnant, you might not have planned this pregnancy, but remember, you made it happen, so get over it and let's start dealing with what you need to know. Don't get all crazy because your friend Jill Jones (the intellectual piranha) read it all in high school before she ever had a sexual encounter, let alone tried to get pregnant. Remember, stop competing and have fun!

If you haven't gotten pregnant yet, but you are biting the bullet to do so, I can help you. Remember, though, sex may never again be as good as it is right now, so enjoy it while you can. Let making a baby be fun; don't make it work, unless of course you absolutely have to. But if you are Type A and you really want to know when to plant the seed, here's how. A relatively normal cycle is on average 25-28 days in length. The length can vary from 21-40 days from the first day of one period to the first day of another. If you want to plan your conception (that is, if you are a career-oriented neurotic who can't just have fun), you will want to keep a menstrual calendar so you know what is normal for you. Also, this calendar will help the physician with determining your actual due date.

In general, the time you will be most fertile is day 10-20 of that cycle, with day 10 being ten days from the first day of your last menstrual period. Therefore, if you have sex every other day from day 10 to 20, a conception should occur in a relatively short time frame. If you want to have sex every night instead of every other, go for it. It won't make his sperm count wither away and die off, nor will it make his sperm too tired to travel the distance. You, on the other hand, might be way too tired to lend a hand in accomplishing this task. Just open up and say "Ahhhh."

The average couple between the ages of 20 and 35 usually takes about six months to conceive. Therefore, rather than work hard at conception, relish the time of being free of worries and concerns about birth control measures. If you are over 35 the likelihood of conceiving quickly is slightly diminished; however, most practitioners understand that you are concerned about your biological clock and will either offer some reassurance or guidance in expediting a conception.

Most physicians are of the philosophy that if a conception doesn't occur after one year of trying, then a thorough workup would be in order. That workup usually starts with a semen analysis.

A lot of men are resistant at first to "put it in a cup," but they tend not to be too hard to convince when their wives say "no cuppy, no nucky." We tend not to put patients through that workup earlier than need be simply because of the anxiety that it can cause the couple.

If you are on the pill and have made the decision to conceive, you should be off the pill for at least one complete cycle before conception. This enables us to better estimate the date of conception as well as decreasing the incidence of twins and pill-related defects. The risk of a developmental defect from the new low-dose pill regimes is no longer of the same clinical concern than it was with the higher-dose pills of the past. Therefore, do not worry if you were one of the few who got pregnant while taking the pill. If you take your pill regularly and do not take any medication that decreases the effectiveness of the pill, the likelihood of conceiving while taking this effective means of birth control is really quite small.

If you are now taking a Depo-Provera shot for contraception and you have made the decision to conceive, we usually recommend that you go off the Depo approximately 3 months (one shot) prior to conception, because the conception rates coming right off the Depo are somewhat slower than off of the pill. If the race is on, remember, coming to the finish line might just take a couple of extra months than it does for your pill-popping friends.

We also recommend that you begin prenatal vitamins prior to conception. Now, if you got pregnant without taking vitamins, please do not worry. Are you worrying anyway? That means you don't have faith in me. Stop that! Relax! Remember, back in the 1600s people didn't have the slightest idea of what to eat in pregnancy, and that was when Sir Isaac Newton was born.

Now I suppose you can make an argument that if his mom ate more seafood he might have been smarter, but jeez, did it really matter that she didn't know all that we now know? I don't think so. And I am quite sure that Einstein's or Beethoven's mom didn't know diddly about the benefits of vitamin B6. If fact, I could guarantee you that Einstein's mom would have never thought that if she'd only eaten more omega-3 fatty acids, her son might have found the answer to immortality and discovered the secrets of time travel.

If you know you are pregnant and have made the decision to learn more, come aboard and we can use this as our starting point. Your conception may have been a boo-boo. So you're not an intellectual piranha or a career-oriented neurotic. You don't have a Type A bone in your wimpy, loony body. But it is never too late to make your body the healthy vessel it was meant to be, for both you and your new passenger.

Now that I hopefully have eased your neurosis, I will tell you that modern medicine does many studies. As a matter of fact, we do studies on top of studies that were already studied. That is by no means a bad thing, but it can make for some confusion, because recommendations seem to be in a state of unending fluctuation. With that being said, I will tell you that as of now, studies have shown that women who are taking prenatal vitamins prior to and during the first months of pregnancy are at decreased risk of their babies developing neural tube defects, such as spina bifida, or problems with the baby's nervous system. That is because the prenatal vitamin has many of the recommended vitamins and supplements responsible for sustaining a good, healthy pregnancy. If you didn't start taking them before, it does not mean you will have a baby with a problem. It just means if you have the opportunity to start before conception, you should do so.

Four hundred mcg of folic acid is present in most prenatal vitamins. It is this supplement that is protective of the developing fetal spine and nervous system and preventative in the formation of neural tube or spinal fusion defects. Research has also shown that vitamin B6 taken before becoming pregnant and during the first few weeks of pregnancy can cause less vomiting and nausea. In an attempt to be proactive, your practitioner will often prescribe these for you when you tell him you are planning a conception. If you choose to use your own over-the-counter supplement, be sure to remember to use a prenatal supplement, because most of the prenatal vitamins are more adequate sources of iron, calcium and folic acid than are the regular daily-allowance-recommended vitamins.

You should look for the following on the label of the prenatal vitamin you choose:

1) at least 4000-5000 IU of vitamin A, and not over 10,000 IU, which can prove to be toxic.

2) at least 400-1000 mcg (or 1 mg) of folic acid

3) no more than 400 IU of vitamin D

4) 200-300 mg of calcium. You should also have a high calcium diet so that you can meet the requirements of the RDA for pregnancy of at least 1200 mg daily.

5) 70 mg of vitamin C

6) 1.5 mg of thiamin

7) 2.6 mg of pyridoxine

8) 2.2 mg of vitamin B12

9) at least 30 mg of elemental iron

10) 15 mg of zinc

11) omega-3 fatty acids and DHA (docosahexaenoic acid), the new up-and-coming supplement of the 21st century, are optional.

The main omega-3 fatty acid is eicosapentaenoic, often abbreviated as EPA. Now, do you really need to know the name of the main fatty acid? No, I don't think so, but some of your friends will know about it. So I am telling you so you won't feel stupid at your next spa day with the girls. The principal source of these fatty acids is marine animals. That is why you have heard so much hype about eating fish and drinking that awful cod liver oil. These marine fatty acids are known to have a protective cardio effect and to be essential to normal neurological development. Preterm birth has also been shown to be less likely in those patients who have a healthy complement of these fatty acids in their diet.

Now I will tell you that if it wasn't for the Internet, these researchers who study all that has already been studied might not have found out about the protective effects of this supplement. How they did acquire such information is quite a miracle, actually. You see, the hypothesis that omega-3 fatty acids could possibly prevent preterm birth was born from studies in the Faroe Islands, which are located in the North Atlantic Ocean between Iceland, Norway, and Scotland. Recorded birth weights on these islands, where fishery is the predominant way of living, were approximately 50,000g, which is on average 200g more than anyplace in the world. Somebody was very bored one day when he used his computer to figure this out. But anyway, he also figured out that gestations were longer by 4-5 days on average. And that is when it happened; they found her off the coast of Norway. *The whale blubber eating lady.*

That's right, you read it right. If it wasn't for her and her obsessive desire to eat whale blubber, the value of omega-3 fatty acids might never have been discovered. The Norwegians, in the course of their studies, discovered a woman whose infants had very high birth weights and who during her pregnancies had experienced an irrepressible craving to consume a traditional Faroese island specialty, blubber from the pilot whale. They also found that the blubber eater had babies that delivered post their due dates. Hence the value of omega-3 fatty acids was further studied, all thanks to her and the poor innocent whales she consumed.

Now, if you are neurotic, you are probably thinking, "God, will I have to eat a whole whale while I am pregnant just so I don't deliver early?" How much fish do we recommend you consume? I can safely assure all of you worrywarts that it will not be a whole whale, nor will you have to eat blubber to get the FDA requirements you need to deliver a healthy, happy baby.

Eating healthy is important in the early trimester and pre-pregnancy time. Most of us know how to eat healthy but use pregnancy as an excuse to gain weight. Some of us eat like pigs normally, but become pregnant and eat like a mega health nut guru. It can't hurt to learn how to eat a healthy complement of foods before you become pregnant. It will not only be beneficial for you and the baby, but it will also help with any undue anxiety you might have regarding your intake of nutritionally sound goodies.

Be cautious in your eating habits. But by all means, enjoy food. I am Italian; I live to eat. That could be why I gained so much weight when I was pregnant. I was raised on macaroni and meatballs. Pasta and fatty meat is not the best combination (not the best in the fatty acid department either, unless lard is someday discovered to be beneficial). Try to tell your 220-pound Italian grandmother that you are eating fish or chicken and salad instead of the Sunday dinner she so lovingly prepared. It ain't easy.

You can treat yourself every once in a while—let's face it, it is tough enough to be pregnant —but think before you plunge into that Sunday sausage, that is all I ask. Try a lean turkey burger instead of a hamburger. If you are not used to eating this way, try it on for size before you get pregnant. Than when you are pregnant, it won't feel like you are torturing or depriving yourself from the foods you are so fond of.

If you are overweight to begin with, we usually recommend that you gain a minimum of 12-15 pounds. On the next page you will find a chart that reviews your BMI (body mass index). Patients like to think in terms of pounds, but doctors like to explain the amount of weight gain by making reference to the pre-pregnancy BMI, which is the ratio calculated based on your weight and height. So if your doctor tells you that you should only gain 15 pounds, then you know you are obese to begin with. If he says you can gain up to 40 pounds, then you are a toothpick and all other pregnant women throughout the world (except in Norway) hate you.

NINE MONTHS TO GO

BMI Before Pregnancy		Recommended Total Gain	
		kg	lb
Low	<18.5	13-18	28-40
Normal Healthy/weight	18.5-24.9	11-16	25-35
Overweight	>25.0-29.9	7-11	15-25
Obese	>30	7	15

BMI

Height (ft-in)	Weight (kg)														Height (m)
	54.5	59.1	63.6	68.2	72.7	77.3	81.8	86.4	90.9	95.5	100.0	104.5	109.1	113.6	118.2	
6'0"	16.4	17.8	19.2	20.5	21.9	23.3	24.7	26.0	27.4	28.8	30.1	31.5	32.9	34.2	35.6	1.82
5'11"	16.9	18.3	19.7	21.1	22.5	23.9	25.4	26.8	28.2	29.6	31.0	32.4	33.8	35.2	36.6	1.80
5'10"	17.4	18.8	20.3	21.7	23.2	24.6	26.1	27.5	29.0	30.4	31.9	33.3	34.8	36.2	37.7	1.77
5'9"	17.9	19.4	20.9	22.4	23.9	25.4	26.8	28.3	29.8	31.3	32.8	34.3	35.8	37.3	38.8	1.75
5'8"	18.4	20.0	21.5	23.0	24.6	26.1	27.6	29.2	30.7	32.3	33.8	35.3	36.9	38.4	39.9	1.72
5'7"	19.0	20.6	22.1	23.7	25.3	26.9	28.5	30.1	31.6	33.2	34.8	36.4	38.0	39.5	41.1	1.70
5'6"	19.6	21.2	22.8	24.5	26.1	27.7	29.3	31.0	32.6	34.2	35.9	37.5	39.1	40.8	42.4	1.67
5'5"	20.2	21.9	23.5	25.2	26.9	28.6	30.3	31.9	33.6	35.3	37.0	38.7	40.3	42.0	43.7	1.64
5'4"	20.8	22.5	24.3	26.0	27.7	29.5	31.2	32.9	34.7	36.4	38.1	39.9	41.6	43.3	45.1	1.62
5'3"	21.5	23.3	25.0	26.8	28.6	30.4	32.2	34.0	35.8	37.6	39.4	41.2	42.9	44.7	46.5	1.59
5'2"	22.2	24.0	25.9	27.7	29.6	31.4	33.3	35.1	36.9	38.8	40.6	42.5	44.3	46.2	48.0	1.57
5'1"	22.9	24.8	26.7	28.8	30.5	32.4	34.4	36.3	38.2	40.1	42.0	43.9	45.8	47.7	49.6	1.54
5'0"	23.7	25.6	27.6	29.6	31.6	33.5	35.5	37.5	39.5	41.4	43.4	45.4	47.3	49.3	51.3	1.52
4'11"	24.5	26.5	28.6	30.6	32.6	34.7	36.7	38.8	40.8	42.8	44.9	46.9	49.0	51.0	53.0	1.49
4'10"	25.3	27.4	29.6	31.7	33.8	35.9	38.0	40.1	42.2	44.3	46.4	48.6	50.7	52.8	54.9	1.47
	120	130	140	150	160	170	180	190	200	210	220	230	240	250	260	
	Weight (lbs)															

Also, most overweight women have at one point or another been on a weight control program or healthy dieting program, whereby they know which foods to eat and which to avoid. However, these usually are the women who tend to use pregnancy as an excuse to pork on the pounds. Therefore, they are also the ones that must be more conservative in their dieting approach. If you are planning your conception and if you are overweight (and who in America isn't?), you might want to exercise. An exercise program can help you lose weight and tone your body in preparation for the challenge of carrying and delivering your baby.

Now if you are very overweight, like 5 foot 2 and 300 pounds, or if your weight is 20% or more over ideal pregnancy weight, your chance of conception might be decreased and you will be at risk for developing more pregnancy-related complication such as hypertension and diabetes. It would also put you at risk for delivering a child who will sustain a shoulder dystocia (a difficult vaginal delivery because the baby's shoulders are too tight to fit under the pubic bone.)

We will talk more about these conditions later on in the book. I mention them now as an early warning, because excess poundage can make you significantly more uncomfortable as you progress in your pregnancy. You might be more susceptible to backaches and varicose veins if you are significantly overweight. If that is the case, and if time is on your side, I do recommend you lose weight prior to attempting conception.

I oftentimes tell my patients not to get too hung up about dieting because it is difficult enough just being pregnant. On average women already think about their weight and dieting just as much as men think about sex. That's about 500 times a day. If you think about it any more than that, you will never get pregnant. Just try your best to eat healthy.

It's important to keep in mind that proper eating during pregnancy is just a matter of common sense. We have an inner ability to recognize what is good for us and what to avoid (unless you live in Norway and like whales). Whether or not we do what is right is a different issue. Obviously, we know to avoid alcohol, tobacco and recreational drugs. We should choose lean meats over fatty ones and low fat milk over whole milk. Broiled food is obviously better for us than fried food.

We want to choose foods that are dense in nutrients and calories, such as dried fruit and nuts. Broccoli and green leafy vegetables are high in vitamin C and calcium. Yogurt and salmon are high in protein and calcium. Yellow vegetables and fruits are very high in vitamin C and iron. Obviously, fresh vegetables are better than frozen and canned vegetables, since they are much higher in vitamins and minerals and much lower in sodium.

It is also very important that our diet incorporates complex carbohydrates as well. This will aid in providing increased amounts of vitamin B and minerals, which will help in fighting the nausea and vomiting that can occur with pregnancy, as well as give us the good calories to help decrease the amount of weight gain. Whole grains, breads, cereals, brown rice, dried peas, beans and potatoes all fit into this category.

If your diet has 300 calories per day more than what is necessary to maintain your body weight, this would be sufficient to gain the appropriate amount of weight in pregnancy. Again, the type of calories is very important; therefore, you should avoid sugary foods. Although aspartame has been proven to be safe in small doses, we do not recommend it as a supplement routinely. If you are in the mood for sugar, we recommend you have fruit juices or juice bars and reserve the sugary foods for special occasions like birthdays, weddings or holidays. Fruit juices, although a good supplement, can be high in calories, so don't drink them constantly. Water should be used to quench your thirst. If you don't like the taste of water or have a hard time getting it all down, use your fruit juice to make it half or quarter strength.

If you feel like snacking, it is more prudent to snack on whole wheat pretzels or toasted sunflower seeds than potato chips or chocolate chip cookies. If you are underweight to begin with, you may take in more than the 300 calories per day that are expected. Also, if you have twins or multiple gestation, you should increase your caloric intake for the amount of gestations that are present, unless, of course, you are having sextuplets, in which case you would need to eat the equivalent of a small buffalo daily to meet your dietary needs.

The amount of protein in your diet is very important. Protein aids in the production of amino acids, which are very important to the baby's growth and development. A decrease in the amount of protein can make for an SGA (small for gestational age) baby. You will require 70-100 grams daily while pregnant. If I have a patient who is also constipated and feeling bloated and unable to eat, I have her make a protein shake with a combination of egg (or if you are worried about salmonella, and you should be if you eat a raw egg, a crushed protein bar would surely suffice), milk, Metamucil, wheat germ and a tablespoon of her favorite ice cream to make it a real frothy milkshake. And then I tell them to get the hell out of town. So far I haven't had any patients complain about this concoction; however, an occasional family member has.

I can't emphasize enough the amount of calcium that is required. Remember that if you are lactose intolerant or you dislike the taste of milk, yogurt, cheese and cottage cheese, which are all high in calcium, then be sure to take your vitamins daily and also supplement with over-the-counter Tums, which are high in calcium. Two Tums per day will be adequate. If you also don't like the taste of Tums, then you are a wimpy whiner and destined to never be happy.

Keep in mind that green leafy vegetables are high in calcium, vitamin A and beta carotene, as well as vitamin E and B6. It is important to have a diet rich in iron, since large amounts of iron are necessary for the development of the baby's blood supply and for your increasing blood volume. Vitamin C is also necessary to aid in the absorption of iron-rich foods. As we already discussed, a certain amount of fat is also necessary in pregnancy. However, remember that too much fat equals excess pounds, and you should have no more than 30% of your calories from fat.

You don't have to worry about you salt intake prior to pregnancy, but you might as well learn how to eat without shaking the shaker, because in pregnancy, salt equals bloating, bloating equals high blood pressure, and high blood pressure can equal pre-eclampsia (toxemia of pregnancy), which can equal your looking like Mimi from *The Drew Carey Show* or Ursula the octopus witch from *The Little Mermaid* (many of you may not be familiar with this character, not as yet having had the opportunity to have a little one watching and re-watching this video over and over again). Therefore, I will re-elucidate, unless you have an overwhelming desire to look like Mick Jagger or a blowfish having a bad day, avoid excessive salt.

Adequate water consumption will be very important when you are pregnant. So it can't hurt to get used to drinking it beforehand. Besides, it is good for you. A rule of thumb is 8x8: Eight glasses of 8 ounces of water per day. This will help to keep your skin soft, decrease swelling, decrease your risk of urinary tract infections, and prevent dehydration, which can be a precursor to preterm labor. It will also keep you extremely friendly with the paper towel lady in the bathroom of the building in which you work. Not to mention that 8x8 glasses of water daily will help you to avoid constipation and, hence, avoid the overabundance of crow's feet and stress lines you might acquire from your exaggerated bearing down efforts. Now we are talking, aren't we? Also keep in mind that if you do a good job of consuming your daily requirement of water, you will be much happier than your cohorts who are not smiling in the waiting room as they sit on their blossoming hemorrhoids.

If you don't feel too thirsty, just try to remember all these positive perks you can receive just from drinking water. Often I have a patient who says she can't drink water because it makes her gag. If that is the case with you, try to mix your water with a tasty fruit juice you enjoy or with Gatorade. Don't just drink the fruit juice or Gatorade in place of the water, because they are very high in calories.

While I do believe that vitamins in no way take the place of a healthy diet, it is still relatively impossible for us to get all the nutrients we need from diet alone, even if your mother is Martha Stewart. Most of us eat on the run and many times are too sick to eat; therefore, it is not realistic to accomplish these dietary goals, so at the risk of sounding like your mother, take your vitamins.

While these supplements are important, they can pose a problem for those of you who have a heightened gag reflex. Oftentimes when you are feeling sick, they are almost impossible to get down. If you take them at night before bed, they are less likely to cause nausea. Remember that nausea is usually present in the first twelve weeks (first trimester) and then tends to subside.

There are many reasons for this. First, the GI tract responds to an increase in the hormone HCG (human chorionic gonadatropin). No, you don't need to know the name of this hormone, but it can't hurt to know that it is responsible for the decrease in bowel motility and the slowing of the bowel's emptying time. This is why pregnant women get easily bloated; food tends to be around a lot longer. The bloating is made worse from the gastric acids that tend to build in response to the stimulus of the hormones. Therefore, when the stomach is empty, nausea tends to be worse.

One solution to this malady is rather than having three normal-sized meals, divide your meals into six smaller ones. If you make sure that complex carbohydrates are a part of each meal, then the amount of nausea will be diminished significantly. In addition, vitamin B6 has been shown to help nausea. If a person cannot take in a sufficient amount in her diet, I do recommend adding it in supplement form. It is sold over the counter in 50-100 mg tablets. Mylanta and some of the other antacids can help greatly in reducing nausea, especially if taken at night, before bed.

It is usually during the night that the gastric acids tend to build up, so that in the morning you might find yourself turning into Linda Blair in *The Exorcist*, ready to paint your room green. Morning sickness is sometimes so severe that people do need to be hospitalized. This condition is called hyperemesis. Women who have this often throw up all day. If their symptoms can't be relieved by prescribed medications, or if the patient cannot self-hydrate during this awful time, then she will need to be admitted and given IV fluids. Luckily, this degree of severity is not common. Most people can find the relief they need in outpatient treatment. Most patients are essentially cured of the condition after the surge of hormones diminishes, which is around the 12th week of pregnancy.

As a resident, I disliked dealing with morning sickness so much, because watching people gag and throw up made me do the same thing. I do think I have a heightened gag reflex, a condition that is not always handy to have as a doctor. I was convinced I would have hyperemesis when I was pregnant. But for some reason I was spared its intensity. I did, however, experience some minor degree of it in waves.

I should mention that morning sickness usually doesn't occur in the morning for most of us, but rather throughout the day. Very often it is worse in those of us who are stressed out, unable to sleep, or not taking in the proper amount of fluids or complex carbohydrates. This is why if you get in the habit of eating properly before you conceive, it might make nausea and vomiting less likely to occur.

If you have a tendency to be seasick, then you will be more likely to develop morning sickness. If you had it in one pregnancy, it doesn't necessarily mean you will get it again. Every pregnancy tends to be different. Nausea usually hits about two weeks after you realize you are pregnant, right around the time when your urinary output increases and your breasts become engorged. The combination of all these factors could make you a real pleasure to be around, as you can well imagine.

Despite the fact that you may be nauseous, you may also develop waves of hunger to the point where if food is not in your immediate reach, you become a wild animal capable of even stealing the Cheerios from your preschooler, who will be left hungry and frightened of your vehement ferocity.

Weighing foods and counting calories in pregnancy is not something I recommend. Just think smart, use common sense, and have healthy snacks available like nuts, grains and granola bars for those real hungry times. And keep away from your poor kid's snacks, for God's sake. Try to take your vitamins, but not to the exclusion of a healthy diet. Once you are pregnant you can always add B6 to your diet if nausea becomes a continued issue.

You could even consider purchasing wrist bands that put pressure on the acupuncture points in the wrist that are supposed to control nausea. If they don't work, they will at least keep your wrists warm in the winter. If you're ever angry at your partner, the wrist bands are nice to throw because they are capable of traveling at great speed and distance due to the metal ball that is used as a pressure point.

If you are a vegetarian, consuming adequate protein can be a bit of a challenge; however, you can certainly maintain your principles and still have a healthy baby. But for those of you who are true vegans, you may have to work a little harder at getting the same amount of protein as your meat-eating, cannibalistic friends. I would also like to let you know how great it is that you are able to maintain this diet without being ravenous. I am a true animal lover. I have tried on numerous occasions to not eat meat. The other sources of protein, however, never seemed to satisfy me. In order to be even remotely satisfied, I had to become a bean-eating bubble of noxious gas. I would float around aimlessly searching for something less combustible to shove in my mouth. I am truly proud of those of you who manage this diet well. And quite obviously, I am not the one who will tell you what you should eat, so I am not even going to try.

If you have had prior medical issues and/or are on medication, you should see your general practitioner before you attempt conception. Changes may need to be made in your medication. Also, pre-conception counseling with a high-risk pregnancy doctor may be helpful. While it is most often not necessary to find an obstetrician before you conceive, you may want to do so in the case of chronic illness to determine how your body might handle the stress that pregnancy may put on you.

Ask your practitioner about the safety of your meds during both preconception and pregnancy. If you have been treated for illnesses in the past such as diabetes, heart disease, high blood pressure and seizure disorders, you may be on a medication that is contraindicated in pregnancy. Also, if a switch in medication needs to be made, it is better to do it before you conceive than to run the risk of having side effects from a new medication in the first trimester. If you are an herbalist and believe herbs can cure you, remember, they can also harm you and may be contraindicated in pregnancy. Be sure to review these herbs with your practitioner.

If you are a smoker, quit. Not only does smoking hurt you and make your lungs black, it also ages your eggs, making it harder to conceive. I don't care about how much it relaxes you or how stressed you are. Chew gum. Smoking does nothing good for you. I just can't comfort you and ease your concerns if you choose to keep up this smelly habit. I guess you know I am a non-smoker; don't hate me if you smoke. I eat instead of smoking, and I probably have a bigger dairy-air than you because of it. But really, it is NOT a good habit!

Is It Done Yet?

Now, let us seriously talk about the various signs of pregnancy. Once you've tried, how do you know you are? If you have been trying and missed a period, I am sure you have done a home pregnancy test—no doubt more than three times. Even though the test showed a positive result, that is, a double line indicating that you are indeed pregnant, or a deep blue positive sign, or better yet, you got yourself one of the new tests out there that say YOU ARE PREGNANT (a pregnancy test for dummies), you will still no doubt wait for your doctor to confirm this rather obvious fact.

The home pregnancy tests can be positive approximately 9-12 days after conception. But rather than spending a lot of time and money in doing a multitude of tests prior to missing your period, it is better to wait until after a missed period, since many obstetricians will not see you for the first 8-10 weeks of the pregnancy anyway. Do you really need to know any sooner? I don't think so. Cool your jets. You are now on the road to changing your life anyway. What difference does 2 or 3 days make?

The reason doctors make the prenatal visit within the 8th to 10th week of gestational age is so that we can assess whether or not it is necessary to perform an ultrasound to determine if your size and dates correspond. We will oftentimes phone in prenatal vitamins when you call for your appointment, that is, if you haven't already started to take them. If you have had a high-risk pregnancy in the past, we will see you sooner. It is important if you chose a new office that you have prior records sent or that you make the office aware of any significant past obstetrical, gynecological or medical history.

The home pregnancy tests are so sensitive that they are almost equivalent to serum testing. But I cannot tell you how many times a patient comes in waiting to hear that she is definitely pregnant from my lips after she has done two, three and sometimes four pregnancy tests at home. Try your best to save money and not be a victim of the insecurity of home testing.

You may be one of the many patients who does not feel that she is truly pregnant until she hears the baby's heartbeat, but believe me, if the test says you are pregnant, then you are. I haven't seen a false positive since the days of my residency, and I won't tell you how long ago that was. The tests nowadays are way too sensitive and accurate to be falsely positive. They may on a rare occasion be falsely negative, but only if done too soon and inadequately.

You might notice certain signs of pregnancy even prior to missing a period. For example, your breasts may become excruciatingly tender to touch, so that even wearing a bra or taking a shower is painful. Once you miss a period, your breasts will continue to engorge. This happens more so in a first pregnancy. I went up three cup sizes with my first pregnancy. But I caution you, don't fall prey as I did to envisioning yourself looking like Jamie Lee Curtis in *True Lies* when she was hanging from the helicopter or like Demi Moore in *Striptease* dancing in front of good ole Burt. You will not become Dolly Parton after you deliver. So don't go changing your career. Those buxom boobs are only temporary.

God plays an evil trick on those of us who are less fortunate. After delivery we not only again return to our original state, but we may possess two very shriveled prunes. So bounce around town with your first pregnancy, ladies, because during any pregnancy after that you will be half the woman you once were. The bottom line is, enjoy it while you can, and don't go purchasing any low-cut dresses too prematurely!

Along with the tender, swollen, sensitive breasts comes a change in color of the nipples and the area around them, called the areola. It is not uncommon for those areas to get deeper and darker in color. Also, people who are naturally dark and have excess pigmentation—you know, those are the ones that tan easily on the beach, while you sit there turning red as a lobster—are the ones who will have the darkest nipples of all. So if you are red-headed and Irish and you just happen to be sitting next to a dark-skinned, beautiful Italian woman in the waiting room of your obstetrician's office, go ahead and laugh at her. You now know that she has some big, bad, black, hairy nipples underneath that cute little pregnancy top she is wearing so gracefully.

As I mentioned, gastrointestinal issues such as nausea may manifest about two weeks after you have missed your period. These nasty symptoms tend to dissipate by twelve weeks, or at the end of the first trimester. But you still may notice prior to that time that you're getting a little more heartburn, and for that reason taking antacids can be helpful. Tums are good for this purpose as they are also high in calcium.

You may also realize that you are belching more. But fear not, you can now go to the zoo on a regular basis and feel safe in the company of animals. At least there the bystanders won't be able to tell the difference between the growl of the tiger and the resounding sound of your belch. You may become much more flatulent as well. And although the antacids may be helping your indigestion, they might take your flatulence to brand new heights. With my first pregnancy I was told by my ex-husband, who had a good but warped sense of humor, that if I could bottle that stuff and sell it to the government, I would make millions! Fear not, Osama Bin Laden.

Although constipation usually develops towards the end of the first trimester, some people may be unfortunate enough to feel the weight of its burdens much sooner. It is caused by the slowing of the GI tract and the weight of the uterus now putting pressure against the lower part of the colon. This condition is enhanced further by the wonderful prenatal vitamins that your doctor prescribed. Therefore, it is essential to take a bulk-forming agent such as Metamucil or Citrucel, which work very nicely in helping the bowels move along more freely.

Because constipation usually makes for very hard stools, this can cause **hemorrhoids**, which can make for very irate patients. Witch hazel soaks or Tucks help make the hemorrhoids retract and can also be very soothing. Over-the-counter preparations with hydrocortisone are safe and can be used, as well as prescription medications. If your 'roids continue to bleed and cause undue discomfort, be sure to make your practitioner aware.

Fatigue is also a very common complaint in the early first trimester. It is not uncommon for a patient to know she is pregnant because of the unnatural degree of lethargy she begins to feel. Some patients are concerned about working through their pregnancies or being efficient at their jobs. Fatigue is not a reason to cut back your work hours; however, use your time at home wisely. Sleep whenever possible. Rest and be a "lady of leisure," allowing others to pamper you when feasible. I was a resident in OB/GYN in my third year with my first pregnancy. Needless to say, when I wasn't working, I was sleeping. I passed out every night on the couch. It was a good excuse not to cook. I don't think I even saw my ex-husband for the first three months of that pregnancy. Turned out that was a good thing for both of us.

Skin changes may occur. Not only may you notice the darkening of the areola, but these areas may elevate. This happens as a result of the hormones of pregnancy. These new bumps on your boobs are tiny glands that help lubricate the nipples. Their perky points come in mighty handy when the baby starts nursing. But for now they are just dark, hairy, ugly protuberances. Calm down.

They will go away, I promise. Most of the time, this discoloration occurs well after the missed period.

You may or may not develop **stria** (stretch marks on the abdomen or breasts). These can occur in the early first trimester, but only if you eat like a hippopotamus. Their occurrence is an event usually reserved for later on in pregnancy. The tendency to develop these lovely, tell-tale marks of our stretching skin is often hereditary, and their size and number are directly related to the amount of weight you gain. Women who gain more than 30 pounds will be more prone to stretch marks. You can't eliminate them no matter what creams you use over the counter. I have patients who bathe themselves in cocoa butter, but if Mom had stretch marks, then they too will develop them. Light-skinned people tend to be more prone to these markings, and although they get lighter postpartum, they never completely disappear. If you have them, don't fret. Consider them battle scars from a war well fought.

You may also get an increased pigment in the line from the pubic bone to the navel area. This darkening again is a result of the increase in the hormone that causes pigmentation. That darn hormone! This begins in the first trimester (when it is not very noticeable) and the line increases for every trimester afterwards. It tends to disappear 3-4 months after you deliver. This is one of the reasons why some doctors may mention to you that sunbathing during pregnancy is not recommended. Besides making you dehydrated, your skin has a tendency to discolor, with an unpredictable pattern of blotching.

You may develop the facial "mask" you may have heard of, which is the pigmented dark skin around the eyes, nose, cheeks and chin. Again, this tends to be a sign that will manifest later in pregnancy. It usually spares the mouth and eyelids, which along with your rapidly growing abdomen is sure to make you look like a panda bear. It is generally more prominent in people who are dark-skinned. Luckily, panda bears are cute and cuddly.

Your History Determines Your Future

Before you actually conceive, you may have many questions about how your past may affect your future. It is always preferable to review your concerns with your doctor, whether they be related to medication or to medical or mental conditions. If you have strict dieting regulations, it may be a good idea to spend some time reviewing with your practitioner ways you can get the proper nutrition for your new addition prior to conceiving, but that is not always crucial.

You may also be wondering what things will soon be like. And I hope to address some of your pre-pregnancy concerns now. But because these concerns tend to blossom as your belly grows, we will reiterate how these potential concerns will affect you at various stages throughout your pregnancy.

Normally your obstetrician will want to see you when you are 8-10 weeks pregnant. Although your initial visit may be scheduled around 3-4 weeks after you call for your appointment, if you are having any problems, such as extreme nausea, pain or bleeding, obviously your practitioner should see you sooner. Be sure also to inform them if you have an obstetrical history that warrants earlier evaluation. If you had a previous elective abortion, you need not see the doctor any earlier, but this will be addressed at your initial prenatal visit. A history of having had a prior **ectopic** (tubal) pregnancy, however, could put you at risk for having another ectopic with this pregnancy, and your doctor might want to see you sooner to obtain the appropriate bloodwork and ultrasounds to rule out this possibility.

If you have never had an ectopic pregnancy before, but you are experiencing any bleeding or pain, then you should make your doctor aware of this as well. Cramping can be very normal in pregnancy. You must remember that the uterus is a muscle, and all muscles stretch and grow. A certain degree of pain can sometimes be associated with this growth. Therefore, menstrual-like cramps are expected and common. Sharp, knife-like pain located in either the right or left lower quadrant, however, can be a symptom of something abnormal.

To make matters more difficult, knife-like pain of short duration can be common after ten weeks' gestation, at which time it may be referred to as round ligament syndrome. This is a pulling of the ligaments that are attached to the uterus and can ache and cause pain with the normal growth of the ever-expanding gravid uterus. Any knife-like pain that increases in intensity, however, and doesn't dissipate quickly should be addressed by your practitioner.

If you have had **fibroids** and they are large and have caused you problems in the past with abnormal bleeding, you should make your practitioner aware at you first prenatal visit. You need not be seen sooner unless you have had prior surgical procedure in an attempt to eradicate these fibroids (a myomectomy). Fibroids rarely prove to be a problem, and many women who are known to have fibroids do carry to term with very few if any complications. Having them, however, can increase your risk of abruption (separation) of the placenta, preterm birth, and a breech lie (the baby being in the foot-down or butt-down position). These conditions are dependent on the size, number, and location of the fibroids.

Where these fibroids are located in your uterus can determine if you may need a C-section. Most of the time fibroids compress easily and therefore do not get in the way of the baby as it comes into the birth canal, but on rare occasions they may block the baby's exit. Painful growth of the fibroids is a rare complication. At your first prenatal visit, discuss the risks of your fibroids with your physician. Every patient's risks are different.

If you have had a prior **second trimester loss** due to an **incompetent cervix**, it is definitely advised that you see your doctor no later than 8-10 weeks, at which time this situation will be addressed. Having had a second trimester loss in the past does put you at risk for another one; however, it does not have to happen again. With careful monitoring and the use of a surgical technique called a **cerclage**, your physician can prevent it.

Any prior loss after twelve weeks, whether second trimester or at term, should be addressed before a conception. Having had the misfortune of such a loss could mean that you have to be treated with baby aspirin or heparin to prevent this rare occurrence from happening again. If you see the same obstetrician as you did with that pregnancy, he will know this and probably will have already discussed it with you and your partner. But if you have switched doctors, you must make your new doctor aware of this prior, very painful experience, and he will need to see you as soon as you have found out you are pregnant so that the proper treatment can be started.

If you are **over the age of 35** you need not see your practitioner before that 8th week, but it is very important that you address prenatal testing and whether or not you and your partner wish to have a more definitive test for chromosomal abnormalities than the noninvasive tests that are currently available. Your doctor will no doubt discuss these options with you at the time of your first visit. The sequential screen that is currently being offered to every pregnant patient regardless of her age is a very accurate screen for such abnormalities, but it is not 100% diagnostic.

We will talk more about this in Chapters 3 and 4, but the current thinking is to not put as much emphasis on being 35 or older. This new thought process does take a lot of pressure off of many women who want to have a baby and have not yet found Mr. Right. So hold on. The clock is ticking a lot slower than it did in 1973. You have time. Don't rush into anything. Having and raising a baby is a full-time job. It is easier to do it alone than it would be to do it with the wrong partner. IVF (in-vitro fertilization) and artificial insemination are options for those of you who really can't find a special enough mate. They are also wonderful mechanisms to aid infertile couples.

Sexually-transmitted diseases can sometimes cause complications during pregnancy and/or delivery, so don't be shy about telling your doctor about your past. There is nothing to be ashamed of. STD's are common, and your doctor can only know what is best for you if you are honest with him. Having had **chlamydia** or **gonorrhea**, for example, may put you at risk for an ectopic pregnancy, because such an infection can increase the chance for tubal disease that may result in scar tissue formation in the fallopian tubes. Alert your doctor and insist on being seen sooner.

Chlamydia is the most common STD and can be passed from mother to fetus. Chlamydia screening is usually done in the first prenatal visit. If you have multiple partners while you are pregnant, you should ask for screening later on in your pregnancy. Once you have conceived, it is not common practice for many obstetricians to inquire about your sexual practices; therefore, to aid in the future health of your baby, be open and honest with your practitioner.

Having had **herpes** in the past does not put you at any risk in the first trimester. You need not be seen any sooner than normally recommended. At the time of your first prenatal visit you must make you practitioner aware of this, however, because antiviral medications will be recommended after 34 weeks. These medications are currently recommended to cut down on the risk of neonatal transmission.

A primary herpetic infection (one that presents for the first time) may put you at risk for a miscarriage if it occurs in the first trimester. If it appears for the first time in the second trimester, it may put you at risk for preterm delivery. And if herpes appears for the first time at delivery, you will need a C-section. A C-section will also be recommended if a recurrence of herpes happens at the time of delivery or in spite of having taken the antiviral medication.

The risk of neonatal transmission is much lower in someone who has had herpes in the past and lower still if that person was treated with antivirals. Having an outbreak at term will require a C-section for prevention, but keep in mind that treatment will help prevent neonatal transmission if that recurrent outbreak goes unrecognized, as it can rarely do. If you have had herpes, you generally will know what to look for, but sometimes patients are asymptomatic shedders. That too is why we recommend treatment if you have a history of herpes. If you haven't had it in the past, you should still make your doctor aware of any lesions you may have that are painful and blistery, as these are infectious for about 7-10 days after they crust over.

Now don't go looking and poking around down there if you are feeling fine. Mirrors are not made for placement in front of your vajayjay. When in doubt, we will check it out. Generally there is no mistaking a first outbreak, because it hurts like hell and usually is accompanied by many blisters.

Don't worry if you are confused by what I've said. I will try to simplify: History of herpes in the past—treat after 34 weeks. Outbreak at time of delivery—C-section. You can ask your practitioner more about it at the time of your first prenatal visit if you have concerns.

Having had **endometriosis** in the past could have been a real pain before pregnancy, but generally it doesn't give you any challenges while pregnant. The biggest hurdle with endometriosis is the infertility and menstrual pain it can cause prior to pregnancy. Now that you're pregnant, you are home free. You are finally going to be symptom-free.

Having taken **birth control pills** and becoming pregnant while taking them (which can happen, but not often) doesn't warrant an earlier visit, but you should stop using the contraceptives as soon as you find out you are pregnant. There isn't any documented evidence of an increased risk of any fetal malformations after having taken birth control pills and stopping them within three months of realizing you are pregnant (especially now with the new low-dose formulas). If you want more information about these and any other potential medication risks, you can go to the pregnancy hotline and website, which will plug in any medication and gladly quote its risks. The toll-free number is 1-888-722-2903, or visit www.snjcp.org.

If you are a DES daughter—that is, your mom took the drug Diethylstilbestrol while she was pregnant with you—this can affect your pregnancy by causing cervical incompetence and the risk of ectopic pregnancy. DES is a drug that was given to patients in the 1950s through the early 1970s to prevent potential miscarriage. If your mom took this drug while she was pregnant with you, you are probably too old to be pregnant now yourself, but if you are, you should make your practitioner aware.

If you conceived by **in vitro fertilization** (IVF), congratulations. The first trimester of this pregnancy will be a little nerve-wracking. The risk of miscarriage is higher in an IVF-conceived pregnancy. More than likely, the infertility (or as they like to be called in the 2000s, *fertility*) docs who took care of you will probably be monitoring you throughout that trying trimester. They will more than likely do frequent ultrasounds to reassure you of the viability of this difficult-to-achieve pregnancy. The doctors will also prescribe the hormone progesterone to help support your pregnancy throughout the first 12 weeks, until the placenta is able to take over the effort of sustaining a healthy pregnancy.

Once the first trimester has successfully passed, you will be sailing smoothly just like everyone else. About 30-35 % of you will be having multiples. If that is the case, the pregnancy will be monitored a little more closely, and you will find out how that pregnancy will be followed as we learn more about what you need to know later on in this book. No more octomoms allowed. Sorry.

Getting **immunized** is always a good idea before pregnancy. If you become pregnant during flu season, we recommend you get vaccinated in the second trimester if at all possible. Live virus vaccines are not recommended during pregnancy. These are measles, mumps and rubella as well as varicella (chicken pox). You can be immunized safely against tetanus, diphtheria and hepatitis B, because these vaccines contain dead or non-active viruses. If you plan on traveling to exotic locations during your pregnancy, you should check with your practitioner to assess whether or not you need to be vaccinated. If you truly have a burning desire to visit with the pygmy tribe of South Africa, try to go before you are pregnant if at all possible.

Dental hygiene is important. Before you conceive, you really want to be sure your gums don't look like you have been enjoying a meal with Hannibal Lecter. It is okay to get your teeth cleaned when you are pregnant, unless you live in Pakistan or Kazakhstan, where many people generally do not brush with toothpaste and those that do brush use dried tree bark. If that be the case, you are more than likely to have infected gums. So for God's sake, clean them before you get pregnant. I mean, do you really want to have breath like a camel?

Having periodontal disease can put you at risk for preterm labor. This risk can be especially heightened if you have always had food between your teeth, and now that you are pregnant, you decide to have a nice pearly-white smile. When at all possible, you want to be sure to keep your teeth clean and not all of a sudden get them cleaned for the first time ever when you are pregnant. You don't want to cause an infection from the disseminated flora that you just decided to attempt to brush away after years of neglect. You should maintain good dental hygiene throughout your pregnancy, and yes, most people can get their teeth cleaned during pregnancy. It is preferable, however, that you get your cleaning before rather than during pregnancy. Keep in mind that your gums will be more sensitive because of the blood flow increase in pregnancy. If your gums are diseased, that sensitivity will be heightened, and some bleeding may occur.

Okay, now that you've tuned yourself up, got your vaccinations up to date, changed your travel plans from Nigeria to New York, took some vitamins, cleaned your teeth, and told your innermost secrets to your doctor, let us move on. But remember, your practitioner is your confidant, and your medical history is very important.

You should be honest and open when asked questions. Your practitioner is there to advise you, comfort you and take care of you without judging you.

Now let's divide pregnancy into trimesters in an attempt to compromise between you and your obstetrician. You as a patient will want to think of pregnancy in terms of months. One of your favorite questions will be, *How many months pregnant am I?* Your obstetrician will want to be in the weekly mode and may even answer your question in terms of weeks. Therefore, we will talk in terms of trimesters since most things happen in threes anyway. You'll find out that most of the things you can expect to occur will be grouped together in periods of approximately twelve weeks, with the length of your first and second trimesters being relatively equal.

Remember, although you will be given a due date (estimated date of delivery or confinement), delivery can occur at term, which is anywhere between 37 and 42 weeks. Preterm is less than 37 weeks. I delivered both of my children at 34 weeks, and considering how much I "loved" my pregnancies, I couldn't imagine going to 42 weeks. Therefore, there are times I find myself more than willing to offer my patients an induction of labor. If I see any medical or obstetrical reason to warrant delivery, if their cervix is extremely ripe and ready, and if I can assure them of fetal lung maturity, than let's go for it is my philosophy. But if my patient would rather trudge along with her big abdomen, backaches and varicosities, more power to her. If you love being pregnant, then you can stay that way until 42 weeks. After that, all bets are off.

To figure out your due date on your own, you can use Nagel's Rule by taking the first day of your last menstrual period, add 7 days to it, then add nine months to it or subtract three months from it, and that is your due date. Or you can just plug your first day of your last menstrual period (FDLMP) into your favorite pregnancy web site.

If you think in terms of weeks (and trust me, you won't unless you are a physician), it is week by week for forty weeks. If you think in terms of months, it is ten four-week months, not really nine months like they make you think. Always remember that the first month really begins seven days after the FDLMP. When you think about it, it sounds kind of weird since you haven't even ovulated yet, but that is the way we docs tend to do it. If you are confused, don't worry, you are not alone.

Just to make it easier for us, so we can rattle off your due date real quick when you tell us you FDLMP and therefore look real smart, we doctors use a pregnancy wheel. These wonderful little wheels not only tell us the date of delivery, but also the probable date of ovulation and where you are in your particular trimester. I think it must have been invented by an overworked obstetrician who didn't feel like figuring anything out at 3:00 a.m.

Now then, just to reiterate, you're in the first trimester from weeks 1-12, or months 1-3. The end of the 12th week begins the second trimester, which starts on week 13. The second trimester lasts from weeks 13-27, or months 4-6. The third trimester starts at the beginning of week 28 and lasts through week 40 (or 42 if you are unlucky enough). The third trimester makes up months 7-9. If you are going to the end of the 9th month, as a patient is occasionally unlucky enough to do, you are actually reaching your 10th month of pregnancy, and God bless you.

Now that we're all on the same track—that is, you went from thinking about it to crossing the line—your life will never be the same. You're done pondering all the what-ifs. You looked too deep into the hole. You fell in, and now, you NEED TO KNOW! Because your breasts are large and tender, your nipples are brownish black and hard, you're nauseous, constipated, and have a headache, let's move on to Chapter Three, "I Got You Babe."

Chapter 3

I Got You Babe

Your First Prenatal Visit

I know you were just thinking about pregnancy and how to prepare your body in Chapter 2, but now you are done thinking and wondering what it will be like. By now you have begun to get a taste of it. Whether you would like to believe it or not, you are pregnant. Your clue may have been a late period or extreme breast tenderness, or perhaps a bout of the uncontrolled expulsion of gaseous contents. Whatever the circumstance that has clued you in… you are here.

Yes, your pregnancy test was unmistakably positive four times in a row, but you still didn't believe it. You did a fifth test and then you decided to call for your appointment. You didn't tell a soul other than your partner simply because you think you might not really be pregnant. The receptionist gives you an appointment for six weeks from now. NO! "I can't wait six weeks to find out!" you yell in the poor girl's ear.

"Honey," she says. "Calm down. If you did a home pregnancy test and it was positive, you are pregnant."

"How do you know?" You are still quizzical and can't dream of telling anyone yet until after you see your doctor. The very next day, after having put your foot in the door with your not-so-sweet phone call, you go to the office of the practitioner you have pain-

Joann Richichi

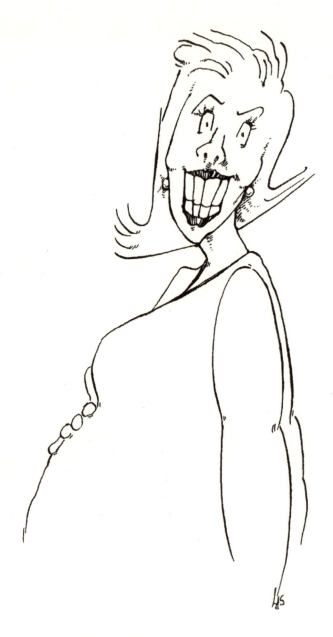

The mask of pregnancy.

NINE MONTHS TO GO

stakingly chosen, ready to harass not the receptionist, but now the nurse. You insist on a serum pregnancy test. Indeed, you are neurotic. But that's okay—you're pregnant and allowed to have periods of neurosis and episodes of irritability and irrational behavior in this, your first trimester.

So finally, after six weeks of waiting to visit your practitioner, you are now about 9 weeks pregnant and it is the morning of your very first prenatal visit. You go to the office and give your name. You tell the receptionist the first day of your last menstrual period. You sit down in the waiting room, look around and see a multitude of different-sized abdomens. The lady next to you is sweating like a pig. The woman across from you is trying to look nonchalant as she sits crocheting while burping incessantly. And somehow there is a familiar aroma that is making your nausea that much worse. Your heart is beating in your ears.

For some reason you're thinking of the movie *Jaws,* and diving into shark-infested waters seems more appealing than what you're doing at present. You want desperately to turn back, but you can't. You know that the inevitable will occur. Your boobs are tender. Your bra is tight. You wish you had a pillow to sit on because you are now paying your dues for eating Nanny's hot peppers the night before. A queasy sensation is tickling your tonsils. The sound of the shark coming to get you in that movie is reverberating in your ears with each beat of your heart getting louder and louder. DA-dun… Da-dun… DA-DUN da-ta da-ta da-ta da-ta- DUN!!!!!!

You're about to wet your pants and there is a line for the waiting room bathroom. Just as you're about to scream, they suddenly call your name. "YES!" you shout as everyone looks at you with sympathy and understanding.

After you have definitely affirmed your presence, you are taken into the office by a friendly nurse, where you will meet with your soon-to-be-enemy, Mr. Scale. You are asked to give a urine specimen, and in your naiveté, you decide to get weighed first. This sequence of events will soon change as the pounds climb; you will choose to empty every orifice prior to your encounter with Mr. Scale. Enjoy him while you can, because soon that metal monster will be called every name imaginable by you. You will realize that the depths of your vocabulary are far beyond your wildest imagination. And don't think that the nurse isn't astute enough to catch on to you when on subsequent visits you decide to take off your shoes. Those visits will be the ones following the weeks when you know that you ate way too much chocolate cake and pudd'n.

The nurse then takes your blood pressure, which is a much less dramatic event than getting weighed ever could be. Then you will be asked to wait in one of the exam rooms, where your doctor will come in to introduce himself to you. You will have a consultation, at which time he will explain to you what your future prenatal visits will entail.

Most patients come to the first prenatal visit with their significant other or partner. This is a very exciting time for couples, and many of them are curious as to what their doctor will be like and how comfortable they will feel with the office staff. Many expectant moms are quite anxious at this time, and their partner tends to allay some of their concerns.

Keep in mind, however, that this visit may not prove as satisfying as you would have hoped. Because this visit is done between 8 and 10 weeks, a small percentage of fetal hearts are actually not going to be heard. We should hear your baby's heartbeat by 11-12 weeks, so don't get discouraged if it is not heard at the first visit. Often times we will have you come back to the office in a couple of weeks, or do an office-based ultrasound or an official ultrasound to confirm that all is well within.

What I am about to review with you regarding the first visit has a lot to do with my experience and my patient population. I will try to address some of the more frequently asked questions that are posed to me during these visits. The questions asked at this early time tend to be more logical and more focused than the ones posed to me later on in pregnancy. I think if given enough time to think, no matter if you are loony or laid back, your imagination can soar. Nine months is a long time to ponder all the "what ifs." During that time, questions may be constantly popping into your head as you experience the pregnancy, along with certain sensations your body is not quite used to. I encourage you to write these questions down so that you don't lose your train of thought between the initial and monthly visits. In the following chapters we will address the other very pertinent questions (and then some) that are asked depending upon your trimester.

I have tried to sum up, in general, when various questions seemed to be posed. Of course, certain issues may present to you at different times in your pregnancy, or hopefully not at all. Just because a patient may have asked me a certain question in her second trimester, it doesn't mean that you have to ask that question to your practitioner in your second trimester. Just be cool, go with what pops into your head and out of your mouth… Maybe if I do my job right, you won't find the need to ask any questions. Boy, wouldn't your doc just love me!

The Consultation

Once I meet the expectant couple, I take them into my office, which is a more comfortable setting. If they are sitting on the examination table while I'm talking with them, they tend to be distracted for obvious reasons. As you might well imagine, it is easier for one to gaze out at the flower bed through the window behind my head than it would be to look at the KY jelly and rectal swabs on the countertop in the exam room. It might be easier to maintain a reasonably comfortable environment by having them read the diplomas and certificates rather than to stare at the Q-tips, single tooth tenaculum and speculum. We mustn't forget to mention the stirrups, which are everyone's favorite part of the gynecological visit.

Once in my office, I then explain to them how I will manage their pregnancy. Provided they don't have any significant medical or psychological issues, I tell them that I will see them monthly, and during those visits I will ask for a urine sample, measure blood pressure and weight, and do an estimation of uterine size. Depending on the gestational age, I may obtain bloodwork and order an ultrasound.

I will also explain that up until 28 weeks we tend to see the patient monthly. After 28 weeks we see them every other week until 36 weeks. From 36 weeks until the date of delivery we see them weekly. This is the standard of care followed by most obstetricians and midwives. Questions are asked and answered; a thorough, in-depth history is obtained. And the dynamics of the practice are reviewed.

A Quick Overview of Prenatal Visits

Generally I finish my consultation before I do the exam, although some doctors do things differently. Once the consultation is over, it will be time to go into the examination room, and although our rooms are meant to be comfortable and homey, we try not to keep patients in this room too long before they meet with us. No matter how comforting the room is, anyone's imagination may stray, and even those of us who have never read Stephen King might be able to write a short story or two reminiscent of his writing style.

An internal exam is done at the first visit before or after the consultation. In general, internals do not usually need to be done again until 36 weeks, unless, of course, the patient has a pregnancy-related complication that warrants an exam sooner. At the 36 weeks a culture will be done for Group B strep, which is a bacterial organism that can cause a potentially harmful infection to an infant delivered preterm, or rarely, to a full-term infant if left untreated. Since beta strep is carried in the vagina asymptotically, a woman would not know that she is a carrier unless we perform a culture, or she had had this bacterium detected during a prior pregnancy.

At 28 weeks a sugar study is done. A woman drinks a sugary drink known as a glucola, and an hour later her blood is drawn. This will assess whether or not the woman has the potential of developing diabetes in her pregnancy. Pregnancy tends to be a diabetogenic state, meaning that if a woman is prone to its development, the pregnancy itself may illicit an unwanted response. It is important for the physician to be aware of this potential, as we will discuss later in the book, since it may require certain treatment in the way of dieting, exercise or perhaps insulin regulation.

Because certain complications are more prone to develop after the 28th week, the physician will see the patient every other week from 28-36 weeks and weekly thereafter. Usually the internals after the 36th week are at the discretion of the practitioner. I personally find very little need to do an internal with every visit. I tend to re-check cervical dilatation and presentation around 39 weeks to assess whether or not the patient may be prone to going post her due date.

I will also reserve my internal exams for those in a lot of discomfort, or those wanting to or needing to be induced. The internal is NOT comfortable. Women are generally engorged and they tend to be hypersensitive (both physically and mentally) at that time. They don't like to be examined unless it is necessary. Some, on the other hand, ask to be examined. Guess who they are? You got it, the career-oriented neurotics! They just gotta know.

The Interrogation

Once your doctor explains how he will manage your pregnancy, he will then ask you a series of questions. Remember, history is very important to the proper assessment of your pregnancy. Be prepared to answer these questions openly and honestly. He will ask if you smoke or if you smoked prior to pregnancy, whether you drink any alcohol or use any recreational drugs, the type of work you do, and the number of hours that you work. While this may make you feel like a spy being questioned about top-secret information, your physician is truly interested in you, and this thorough history will help him better predict the outcome of your pregnancy. The inquisition will enable him to detect and treat you early for potential complications.

Your physician might ask, "What pregnancy is this for you?" You might have had an abortion and you might want to lie and say the first, but you should tell the truth. One or two abortions would not make a major difference to this particular pregnancy, but having had five or six could result in a situation in which the cervix may become incompetent or less able to support the pregnancy. You need to let him know the timing of that prior abortion; for example, if done in the first trimester, the abortion is not likely to have any impact on this or future pregnancies, but if done after the 14th week, and if you had more than two abortions done around that time period, you might be at slightly increased risk of premature delivery with this pregnancy.

If you tell him that you haven't had any prior pregnancies, the rest of the history-taking regarding prior pregnancy-related issues will be over. However, if you have had any prior pregnancies, he will want to know the details of those pregnancies, such as whether or not they went to term, what the birth weights were, their sexes, whether or not they were delivered spontaneously or if they required the use of vacuum or forceps.

If a C-section was done, he will want to know why—was it a big birth weight baby? Did you progress to a certain centimeter dilation? Was there an element of fetal distress, or did you have a pregnancy-related complication necessitating a C-section, like high blood pressure or severe pre-eclampsia? Did you have any gestational diabetes with that pregnancy, which would make you prone to its reoccurrence in this pregnancy?

He will also want to know if you have had any prior gynecological problems, such as infertility, whether or not you conceived on any fertility drugs, and if you have had any gynecological surgeries in the past. He will ask if you have ever had abnormal pap smears or fibroids (benign growths) in your uterus. You will also be asked if you have been subject to frequent urinary tract infections or to sexually transmitted diseases, or if you have been exposed to hepatitis or AIDS or had Group B strep.

He will want to know if you have had any hospital admissions for chronic lung disease, asthma, bronchitis or heart disease, such as congenital defects, rheumatic fever or mitral valve prolapse (MVP). He will also want to know if you or your partner has any family members with congenital defects of any kind, since these can be hereditary. For example, having a nephew with a congenital heart defect can be a hereditary occurrence, and your practitioner should be made aware.

He will want to know if there is any mental retardation or history of chromosomal abnormalities in either family. And he will also need to know if anyone in your family has hypertension or diabetes, which may make you more prone to the development of these diseases while pregnant. He will ask if you have any nutritional concerns with your diet, such as whether or not you are a vegetarian or whether or not you avoid certain foods on a regular basis.

He will inquire about your genetic background to see if your child could be affected by certain hereditary disorders such as Tay-Sachs disease, which is a concern if you are of Jewish descent, or sickle cell if you are of African-American descent. Each of us may carry a gene for a genetic disorder, but most disorders need a matched pair of genes to cause a disease in an individual.

If there are any particular concerns, one or both parents can be tested for some of these disorders before or during the pregnancy. We don't test everyone because the testing does not make sense unless there is an above-average possibility that both parents are carriers. That is why ethnic or geographic questions may be posed. It is not because your doctor is a nosey bugger, although it might seem that way at first.

For example, we now test everyone for cystic fibrosis, or CF. The gene for CF is carried by 1 in 25 Caucasians. Because we can never know for sure who married who way back when, we test everyone. Jewish couples whose ancestors came from Eastern Europe may carry Tay-Sachs or Canavan disease. If both of you are not Jewish, we will not offer the testing. If you are Mediterranean and Asian, your doctor may want to check for thalassemia or other hereditary forms of anemia. In most cases, the testing is recommended for one parent: that would be you, our patient. Since we are drawing your blood at this visit to obtain your routine labs, we might as well get the whole dang thing. Your partner gets off easy AGAIN!

While we are talking about genetics, it is now the time to fess up if you married your first cousin Billy Bob. Closely related couples risk inherited disease in their offspring. If this is the case, or if any hereditary issues are posed, your practitioner will send you for genetic counseling. Seeing a geneticist prior to becoming pregnant is always recommended in the case of any familiar hereditary issues, because the counselor is trained in giving the couple the odds of their having a healthy child based on their particular genetic profile. They are the ones who can guide the couple as to whether or not they should even have children to begin with. But don't worry, because meeting with the counselor even after you have become pregnant can be most helpful. Along with the high-risk pregnancy doctor, the counselor can outline all the options available and help the couple decide how to best proceed with this particular pregnancy.

You will be asked if you have any allergies to any medications. And on a more personal level, your doctor will want to know if you have any psychosocial issues that may prove to be stress-producing throughout your pregnancy, other than the fact that you married Billy Bob, that is. And if he does not ask, because there is so much to ask and certain questions may unintentionally be overlooked, please tell him about anything that may be weighing heavily on your mind.

NINE MONTHS TO GO

It Gets Worse—The Exam

As mentioned, the very first prenatal visit, in addition to the question-answer consultation, will include an exam to determine the size of the uterus and, therefore, to see whether or not the dates of your FDLMP and probable conception adequately correspond to the uterine size. If they do, than an early ultrasound need not be performed. However, if the size is bigger or smaller than the dates given by the patient would suggest, the physician may order an ultrasound, since one done early in gestation is more accurate in determining the proper dating of the pregnancy. A first-trimester ultrasound can also confirm the viability of the pregnancy and determine the number of fetuses, especially if there is a size-date discrepancy.

As of the year 2008 we offer everyone a first-trimester combined screening along with a second trimester ultrasound assessment of fetal anatomy. The days of only doing the non-invasive quad screen test for chromosomal abnormalities, which so many of you have heard of, and perhaps even have had in prior pregnancies, is now coming to an end, being replaced with newer and more accurate screening. Modern medicine and technology never ends, does it?

We will talk about this in more detail when we discuss maternal testing after the exam section in this chapter. But keep in mind that these tests are offered as an assessment of fetal well-being. If at any time along the course of our thorough investigation they show a problem, then we can offer you further invasive testing, such as a CVS (chorionic villus sampling) and amniocentesis, which unlike the screening tests, are diagnostic and can tell you with 100% accuracy whether or not you will be having a child with a chromosomal abnormality. Keep in mind also that if you are over the age of 35, you are given the opportunity to have a diagnostic test regardless of the results of your sequential screen. In other words, if your screen gives you reassurance, but you need to be 100% sure of your baby's chromosomal status, you can opt for more. Since Down Syndrome can also occur in mothers under age 35, everyone is entitled to the option of invasive screening. But, as the word "invasive" implies, there are risks that may outweigh the benefits of diagnostic testing. This is why screening is a good option for women under 35.

A second trimester ultrasound, or anatomy scan, as it is often called, is the standard of care and every pregnant patient will be given one. The maternal-fetal medicine specialist or perhaps the radiologist can at this time more accurately assess the fetal spine, brain, nervous system, heart and other organs.

The issues and questions surrounding tests, and which ones to perform at which time in pregnancy, can get confusing. I want to put a lot of time into explaining these tests in a clear, less perplexing manner. I want to limit what you need to know. I could write a book about this topic alone, and I really don't think you need to know all the details about the new and improved tests that are offered. You just need to know whether or not you want to have them done, and if so, which ones you feel comfortable with having. Insurance shouldn't be an issue, because this testing is now offered to all as a standard of care. If in the next section you find that I don't cover it in enough detail for you, than go ahead and make yourself crazy and search the Internet. You deserve to get what you're in for.

At the time of the first exam, the physician will also obtain a pap smear and a cervical culture for chlamydia, which is an organism that can be sexually transmitted and is the most common infection passed from mother to fetus. Because this infection can be a possible risk to the fetus, chlamydia screening is done on all pregnant patients. So don't get insulted if you have been married to your husband for the last ten years and we want to test you for an STD. We are not accusing any one of infidelity; we are concerned about your *bambino*—we are not calling you a *bimbo*. We simply need to be sure that your baby is not at risk for developing an eye infection or pneumonia as a result of this disease, which may have been asymptomatic in you but can be passed to your newborn. Although the best time for treatment is before conception, infected pregnant women can be treated by simply administering oral antibiotics (usually azithromycin) to them.

The antibiotic ointment routinely placed in the baby's eyes at the time of birth protects the newborn from chlamydial and gonorrheal eye infections. Although gonorrhea is less common, it has been the culprit in neonatal conjunctivitis and blindness in fetuses delivered through an infected birth canal. For this reason, all pregnant women are routinely tested at their first prenatal visit. If you are at high risk for STDs (and you know who you are) you should ask to have the test repeated in late pregnancy. Treatment is instituted at the time of a positive culture. The culture is rechecked several weeks later to be sure that the woman is free of infection.

Once the cultures and the pap are done, the practitioner will do a bimanual exam, the same one that is routinely done at the time of your annual visit. That is when he examines your uterus with his hands to determine its actual size. No, his whole hand does not go into your vagina. He uses the two fingers of one hand inside the vagina and the four fingers of his other hand on the super pubic area of your abdomen, where he will press down on your abdomen in an attempt to estimate uterine size.

During this first exam, if the uterus is felt to be much bigger, it can mean that the dates are off. It can also mean that you are having twins or that you have a fibroid. If the uterus is found to be much smaller than expected by the physician, it could mean that your dates are off, or that you may have sustained a type of miscarriage called a missed abortion, meaning that you didn't bleed yet, but that the pregnancy did not progress as it should have. It also may signify the potential of a tubal (ectopic) pregnancy, or perhaps a less worrisome scenario such as your uterus being retroflexed, meaning angled posteriorly, so that the physician cannot feel the total extent of the uterus.

Although we are currently recommending and offering sequential screening, which begins around week 11-14 with an ultrasound and bloodwork, your doctor may order an ultrasound to be done sooner, prior to the one done at the time of your early screening. If he orders an ultrasound, realize that it is only done to better affirm the accuracy of the pregnancy. Don't panic. Understand. While it is good to know the various possibilities, have trust in your physician; he is trying to verify and rectify the situation if need be.

Prenatal bloodwork will also be ordered. Many physicians do the bloodwork in their office, but some will send you to a local lab to have it drawn. A blood test to determine your blood type and Rh status will be done. Occasionally an HCG level will be done to assess the viability of the pregnancy, especially if you have had any first trimester bleeding. The bloodwork will include a CBC (blood count), a hepatitis screen, and an HIV test with your permission. A test for syphilis will also be done, although this infection is much less common than it was in the '70s and '80s.

In addition to that, depending on the type of work you do, your physician may order tests such as a CMV titer (cytomegalovirus) and/or a parvovirus titer (fifth's disease). For example, if you are a daycare worker, you're more prone to be around children who carry these viruses. Also, if you are a nurse or health care provider, CMV can be contracted through patient care. Most of us do have antibodies because many of us have had the virus as children. Sometimes reactivation can occur, and if so the virus can be transmitted to the baby, but is less likely to be. If you are in this line of work it is important that you wash your hands frequently, and be sure to ignore your boogers until you can blow hard or use a Q-tip. Picking your nose is a definite no-no!

Parvovirus is also called B19 virus or fifth's disease (it has more names than my Aunt Tootie) and is the fifth out of six commonly occurring viruses caught by children. The child may experience a reddish glow in the cheeks, cough and runny nose. As an adult you may not experience any symptoms, but the virus can prove harmful if contracted in the first trimester, when it can be a rare cause of miscarriage and fetal anemia.

You will have genetic testing for CF and, if appropriate, you may also have genetic tests for sickle cell anemia and Tay-Sachs, as we have discussed. A hemoglobin (HAIC) may be obtained to assess if your sugar has been adequately controlled prior to pregnancy, especially if you have a family history of diabetes, have high blood pressure or have had a previously large birth weight baby.

If you have a household cat, a toxoplasmosis titer may be ordered. Most people who have had cats for some time do have antibodies to this infection. Most of us have already been exposed. The exposure doesn't have to have been from your poor, innocent cat either. Eating raw meat (you animal) or drinking unpasteurized goat's milk can also be the culprit. Tell me, who drinks goat's milk? With all the milk products out there—Lactaid, soy, low-fat, no fat —why goat's milk? If you are a goat milk drinker, call me, e-mail me... I just want to know why.

Most of us docs do not do regular testing on all those who have cats since most have the antibodies. Testing is most warranted if you have never had a cat and all of a sudden you decide to get yourself a brand new baby kitten. Or you have an overwhelming desire to adopt some full-grown cats and now are the owner of some new indoor-outdoor pussies when up until this point you never had a cat to love and to cuddle. But even though we may choose not to test you, we ask that you take some precautions:

1) We would encourage you not to change the litter throughout your pregnancy, and wear gloves if you must do this task. You may now easily assign this task to your partner, but he will probably never do it and you will wind up having cat feces throughout your house because the poor cat can't even fit in his litter box. By not being so compulsive about sifting through the litter box yourself, however, you will lessen your exposure to the toxoplasmosis *gondii oocyst*, which is excreted in the feces of the infected cat.

2) I personally love cats, but I discourage my cat from sticking his butt in my face. I only ask that you do the same. Be affectionate with your feline pals, but remember that the oocyst which causes the infection is located in Felix's little anus. So when your perfect little pussy stretches and struts her derriere between your eyes, remember to look the other way. And by all means, don't breathe.

3) Don't eat raw meat, and if you have the desire to eat a steak, cook it, for God's sake. I mean, what are you, a cannibal or something?

4) Use gloves when you handle raw meat.

5) Wear gloves when you garden because the soil may have cat deposits in it.

6) Wash all your fruits and vegetables. (Do I sound like your mother or what?)

    I think that about covers the blood tests that we routinely do with your first visit. It doesn't cover that sequential screen and integrated screen I spoke of. You will have to come back for that if it is available in your facility, or you will be sent to a local high-risk specialist if you choose to have it done. Don't worry, we will get to all that. I am just saving the best for last.

    In addition to these blood studies, a lyme titer should be done if you live in a heavily wooded area or do a lot of gardening, if you are a veterinarian or vet tech, or you work with animals. Lyme is particularly prevalent in New Jersey. Having been a victim of this insidious illness, I tend to be very liberal in obtaining titers on my patients. Lyme can cause complications such as fetal anemia and preterm birth if left untreated.

    Don't forget to pee-pee before you sneak out the door. The reason your physician will want a urine specimen at every visit is because urinary tract infections are very common in pregnancy, and most of the time they are silent since the frequency and urgency caused from pregnancy itself tend to mimic the symptoms of a urinary tract infection. Approximately 20% of the time the urinary tract infection can result in a kidney infection, especially if left untreated or undiagnosed. They are easily treated with antibiotics.

It is very important that you stay well hydrated and that you keep the vaginal area clean, and always make sure that your bladder is empty. Sometimes it may prove difficult to completely empty your bladder, especially in the late second trimester when the baby's head tends to impinge against the bladder, causing a funneling of the fluid. A way around this is after you void, turn around, stand up and lean forward, pressing a hand against your pubic bone so as to further empty your bladder. I caution you—you're safe if you do this in a coed bathroom, but if anyone witnesses your feet facing the other way in the stall of a ladies' bathroom and they hear the tinkle of your urine, they may believe that you're packing more in those pants than just your expanding abdomen.

Okay, folks, now for the confusing part. Everyone is offered a form of genetic screening. There are multiple reasons for offering this, mainly that most of us like to know what to expect. It wasn't enough to have this information available to us in the second trimester with the ultrasound and quad screen we offered all our patients up until a year ago. The second trimester was too late to do something about the chromosomal situation if someone chose. So came the new and improved first-trimester assessment.

I would just like to say before I begin this segment that I have many patients with children who have Down syndrome. I am both thrilled and amazed at how many of these patients consider these children a profound gift from God. I can see how happy they are and how their lives have been blessed. But many consider the possibility of having such a child in their lives a potential burden to life's already difficult and sometimes tortuous road. This screen offers those a way to find out and either prepare for the outcome or terminate its potential.

For more information regarding this difficult personal decision, I refer you to the list of "Books for a Down Syndrome Pregnancy" at the end of this chapter. Perhaps the experiences of others will help you to understand more about Down Syndrome and what it can mean for you and your family.

Quad screening is a blood test that measures the levels of four substances that are passed into the mother's blood and are produced by the growing fetus. This is done through one simple blood test performed on the mother between weeks 14-21. The substances tested in the maternal blood are alpha fetal protein (AFP), HCG, inhibin-A and estriol. Up until five years ago a triple screen was done instead, which only tested for three of the substances. To make things more confusing, if a patient opts for diagnostic testing instead of screening, a quad screen need not be performed and a triple screen will be recommended instead in the second trimester. It will be done around the same time that the anatomy scan is offered.

High levels of AFP may suggest that the baby is at risk for neural tube defects, while low levels may indicate that the baby is at higher risk of chromosomal abnormalities, specifically Down syndrome. Down syndrome is the most common cause of severe learning disabilities in children. It occurs in about 1 of every 700 births. Down syndrome is also called trisomy 21. Its occurrence is not preventable. Those at most risk—or as some of my patients might say, those that are most likely to be blessed by having a child with this condition—are

1) Older women (over 35)

2) Parents who have had a baby with either Down syndrome or another chromosomal abnormality.

3) Those with siblings or first degree relatives with Down syndrome.

Testing can be done at the end of the first trimester and/or the beginning of the second trimester. The more accurate test is one that uses information from tests done during both the first and second trimesters (called integrated testing). First the ultrasound is used to measure a thin layer of fluid that accumulates in the back of the baby's neck. This is referred to as nuchal translucency (NT). Increased fluid may indicate an increased risk of chromosomal abnormalities such as Down syndrome. The blood test done at the same time measures levels of PAPP-A (pregnancy associated plasma protein A) and HCG. These levels, combined with the NT and the mother's age, can provide a risk assessment for Down syndrome and trisomy18.Combined screening can't give you a definite diagnosis, but it can help you decide whether to get more diagnostic tests. An elevated maternal serum alpha-fetal protein (MSAFP) can tell the doctor if there may be a future problem with the growth of the baby that could necessitate an earlier-than-expected delivery.

If the screening tests show an increased risk, you can opt for CVS or amniocentesis, or you can move on to the second half of the screening assessment, **integrated testing**. This is done in two parts. The first part is done in the first trimester and includes the ultrasound and the PAPP-A. The second part is done at 15-20 weeks and includes the quad screen. The results of the first and second parts are integrated (combined) to give a single number that estimates the fetus's risk of having Down's. This will be reported after the second trimester testing is completed. It identifies 85% of women carrying a baby with Down's. Only about 1% of those screened have a false positive result. Integrated screening can also be useful if early ultrasound is not readily available, or if the fat pad on the back of the baby's neck cannot be seen because of the baby's position or the mother's weight.

The disadvantage of this mode of combining the testing is that information is not provided until later in the pregnancy (typically after week 16). That is why there is **contingent sequential testing**. This process involves having the results of the first trimester portion of the integrated screen reported immediately, with the next step being dependent upon these results.

If the test shows that the woman is at very high risk of having an affected fetus (1 in 50), then she could elect to undergo a CVS, or an early amnio. If the screen shows the woman to be at very low risk (1 in 2000), then no further testing is necessary. In this population we still offer quad screening and an anatomy scan to everyone. That is the difference between contingent and just plain old sequential screening.

If our perinatologist (maternal-fetal specialist) feels that further testing is recommended to give more accurate reassurance to the expectant parents, regardless of the reassurance given with the first portion of the screen, we perform the second section as well. If the first trimester portion of the screen is reassuring, then your practitioner may recommend the quad screen in the second trimester. If the test shows the woman is at intermediate risk (between 1 in 50 and 1-2000), then she would complete the second trimester portion of the blood test (integrated). Now you are in the second trimester and CVS is no longer an option, but amniocentesis is.

So then, when are these tests recommended and for whom?

1) If a woman wants to know her risk as early as possible.

2) If a woman prefers to avoid a diagnostic test, the integrated screen is recommended.

3) Even in someone who would not consider terminating, we still recommend the screening process to learn about the baby's risk of birth defects. Having the knowledge can help the couple and medical team better prepare for the baby's birth.

4) For an average-risk woman who would want to consider terminating her pregnancy if her fetus had Down Syndrome, first trimester testing, whether it be integrated or sequential, is definitely recommended.

5) For a high-risk woman who would not consider terminating but wants to know, integrated or sequential testing is recommended. That woman could then choose to have diagnostic testing. Keep in mind that if a CVS is performed, the patient will still be offered a second-trimester MSAFP as a further assessment of fetal well-being.

If you live in the boonies, this new improved means of testing may not be available. The perinatologist or high-risk pregnancy doctor is usually the one who performs and reviews the ultrasounds for NT. If this is not offered at your facility, don't worry. The quad screen and ultrasound in the second trimester worked well enough in the past, and I am sure your practitioner will offer you what he feels is appropriate for your pregnancy. What you choose to do with that is totally up to you. Remember, it is your pregnancy and your future. All we can do is hope to inform you well so you can make a decision as to how you wish to proceed. Most of my patients opt for the sequential screen regardless of their age. In actuality, many more babies with Down Syndrome are now born to women under 35, which is why the testing is offered to all women regardless of age. Keep in mind that the advantage of *screening* is that it is non-invasive. It will NOT tell you for sure if the baby is "affected," but will tell you if the baby is at higher risk for chromosomal abnormality.

Okay, enough of that! Now let's move on to questions you might ask at this visit. Now that your doctor has spent the last 15 minutes talking about the damn testing, you not only don't feel like asking questions, but you've forgotten what the heck you wanted to ask. Or you might remember what you wanted to ask, but you are so damn sick of him talking you just don't want to ask anything. Even so, you might be wondering about these things anyway. Hopefully I will answer for you those questions you meant to ask but just couldn't at the end of your first prenatal visit. Here goes.

FREQUENTLY ASKED QUESTIONS—
IT'S YOUR TURN!

How much weight should I gain? or **How did I gain so much weight already? I hardly ate anything.**

I tell patients that I like them to gain between 22-28 pounds. In actuality, anywhere between 25-35 pounds is appropriate. Many of the books that patients read will tell them that it would be more prudent to gain one pound per week from week 8-32, with 3-4 pounds being gained in the first trimester, one pound per week in the second trimester and approximately one pound per week in the third trimester, and only 1-2 pounds in the ninth month. Now I don't know about you, but it's hard enough to know that you have to gain 25-35 pounds. Knowing *when* you have to gain it is a whole different issue. I tell my patients to gain weight at a steady pace, never to lose weight and never to diet.

I tend to be somewhat strict with women who gain an excessive amount of weight early on, since I porked out at a whopping 42 pounds with my first pregnancy and 37 pounds with my second. I had the excuse of preterm labor and bed rest, but being only 5'1", I had a lot of work to do after delivery to get back to a relatively respective figure. Every pound over 30 seems to be difficult to lose and can be a true reason for a woman's experiencing postpartum depression.

Staying in the weight gain range of 22-28 pounds will help in avoiding a difficult vaginal delivery. If you are very overweight to begin with and concerned about the amount of weight you may gain with this pregnancy, your doctor may encourage you to gain only 12-18 pounds. Although the baby's size is genetically determined regardless of weight gain, too much weight gain can result in a very large baby, which can make for a difficult vaginal delivery and a condition known as shoulder dystosia, which we'll talk about later. Avoiding excessive weight gain can also prevent the increase in varicose veins, pelvic vein engorgement and pressure that some women are unlucky enough to experience.

It is not prudent to carefully weigh everything that you put in your mouth; just think in terms of healthy eating. Remember that the middle of the second trimester to the 34th week of the third trimester is when the fetus has an acceleration in its growth and, therefore, this is when the calories are used most efficiently and weight gain is most effective. If, however, you gain too much in the first trimester, you still need to go ahead and increase the weight at a steady although slower rate. Although babies do take what they need from your accumulated fat stores, it is important that you meet the necessary nutritional requirements so that you don't become depleted.

If you gained a lot of weight in the first trimester, it's going to make it more difficult for you in that you're going to have to concentrate on the type of calories that you're eating in the second and third trimester. If you do that without gaining a lot of weight, most physicians will be satisfied that you are slowly increasing weight without packing on the pounds. Don't worry, if you failed in the first trimester you won't have to look like a sumo wrestler in the third trimester in order to have a healthy baby. The reason you already gained a lot of weight is not because you are going to have a big baby, it is simply because ever since you found out you were pregnant you have been eating like a little piggy. Slow down. We have nine months to go, for goodness' sakes.

I have headaches when I'm not pregnant; will they get worse when I'm pregnant? Or, I have migraines. What will I be able to take for them?

Headaches can and often do worsen in the second trimester from hormones that are increasing and fluctuating throughout the pregnancy, in addition to the increased blood volume that results in vascular dilatation. If you are suffering from headaches, you will be more likely to have fatigue and physical and emotional stress as a result of them. You can treat them with increased fluids and Tylenol. You can take as many as two Tylenol every four hours if necessary, even Extra Strength Tylenol. If you find you need more than this, contact your practitioner. Every drug has its risks if taken in excess. Although it is very rare, liver toxicity can occur with overuse of Tylenol. Most things are fine, though, if done in moderation.

You should *not* take any aspirin derivatives, Motrin or Advil. If you are prone to migraines, there are medications that can be used in pregnancy if they do become severe. You should, however, speak to your family doctor or neurologist, who will work with your obstetrician in this regard.

Can I have sex?

My answer is, most definitely YES! Unless, of course, you are in the first trimester and bleeding, or if you are closer to the end of your pregnancy and have a history of having preterm labor, a placental abruption or a placenta previa (when the whole placenta or a piece of placenta covers the cervix or the opening of the womb). Orgasm can result in uterine contractions, which can increase the likelihood of a preterm delivery. So if you are being treated for preterm labor or you are at risk for it because you had it with a prior pregnancy, then you will have to restrain yourself.

In addition to the mighty O being a potential problem, the almighty sperm can be a culprit in cervical dilation and effacement because of its high concentration of prostaglandins. Prostaglandins are used to effect cervical effacement (the thinning out of the cervix) for people who need an induction of labor for various medical or obstetrical concerns or complications. Prostaglandins are carried in the head of the sperm. A high concentration of sperm in the vagina from an ejaculation can result in cramping and discomfort. Who said that men didn't have important assets in those little heads of theirs? If you do complain of a lot of cramping post-intercourse, your doctor may suggest withdrawal and/or the use of condoms. No, he is not suggesting this because he is a mean man.

Therefore, having sex excessively can result in preterm labor. What is excessive? It depends on who you ask. But if you can keep it to less than three times a week, you should be okay. Also remember that if sperm is not involved in your lovemaking, you can probably get away with more than that. But you are pregnant, for God's sake; do you really want to have sex that much? If you do, more power to you. What do I know? I am almost menopausal now. I forget what it was like to be young and horny, but that is another book for another time.

Some patients (the lucky ones) tell me that they are extremely horny while pregnant and want to have sex all the time. They actually want to know if too much nucky can hurt the baby. If their faithful partner is present, he may ask if he will hit the baby's head. Is that guy on an ego trip or what? Number one, you won't hurt the baby, and number two, unless your partner is Bigfoot or has a willy the size of a bull's or elephant's (1½ feet average length), he won't hit the baby's head no matter how hard or what position he may pursue.

Most pregnant women have an increased libido in the early part of pregnancy when their labia are engorged from the increased vascular dilation. Towards the end when they have a bulging abdomen looming over their hidden valley, most women feel it's just not worth the trip of going around the mountain. Others, however, look at this time as an adventurous endeavor of experimenting and finding new positions. Who said size doesn't matter!

The increased engorgement and lubrication that occurs in the first trimester can prove to be a source of enjoyment for most women. It may heighten their sexual response. On the other hand, it might cause their partners to slide right out of town. The swollen labia may cause a woman never to quite climax, but always to be on the plateau. Don't fret—at least you're being intimate, and considering how beautiful you now feel, that's quite a feat.

Enjoy sex, enjoy the intimacy, but don't make having the "big O" your number one goal. It's finally a time when you don't have to worry about the restraints of birth control, the difficulty of having to conceive, or the possibility of being infertile, and it is a time to be free of inhibitions. It's not uncommon for both partners to experience a wide swing of emotional disturbances when they come to the realization that they will no longer be just lovers, but also parents.

Does the baby know when we are having sex?

Yes! The placenta has a built-in observatory for your child to gaze at his father's dick as it hits the opening of the womb in which he is being held captive. Now really, folks! I don't care what you think, you are a true neurotic if you are worried about this. For those of you who are apprehensive that your infant could be watching or experiencing the sexual act with you, think about this: when was the last time you heard of some kid talking to his parents about what their sex life did to him while he was in utero? If that were the case, the shrinks would have a heyday treating neurosis caused by intrauterine sex-induced stress—and believe me, it would have been on Oprah.

When my partner manipulates my breasts, I feel cramps. Is that normal?

In the second trimester your newfound toys may become so perfectly perky that your man may not be able to keep his hands off them. You, too, may have a new zest for life, but be careful—your excitement will be short lived. As you progress in pregnancy, not only will your playing with these cause leaking and irritation of the nipples, but it can cause contractions, which then can cause the letdown of milk and also preterm labor. Therefore, remember that anything in moderation is okay, but proceed with caution. Overuse and abuse can prove harmful to your health. Life can be cruel.

NINE MONTHS TO GO

I'm afraid of stretch marks. What can I do to prevent them?

Well, 90% of women do get stretch marks. They can lighten up following a pregnancy approximately 3-4 months later. You can accelerate the decrease in tint by applying vitamin E in various oils. However, it also depends upon the amount of weight that you gain. There is a strong hereditary potential, and if you are prone to them, regardless of your weight, you will get them. You can minimize them with exercise and proper nutrition and hydration.

My mom had horrible stretch marks. I remember looking at her abdomen when I was a kid and saying, "My God—how could having a baby be worth those things?" I was so fearful that I too would have them. Luckily I never got one. But then again, I never got her 36 DD's, and they're supposed to be hereditary too! I definitely took after my father when it came to that.

Being in practice for ten years now, I am still often amazed at the type of questions that I am asked. One of the questions I have gotten in the past I'm convinced I have gotten only because I am a woman (sometimes I do envy my male colleagues), and believe me, I have gotten this question more than once. Are you ready?

I have vaginal farts when I have sex. Is there something wrong with me? Is the baby getting air blown into his head?

(And this is what I went through medical school to answer!) It may seem silly as you read these words right now, but believe me, the women who asked this question were sincerely worried and frightened. Fear not, I want to tell them. If you're having "vaginal farts" now, wait till you push this 10-pound joy out of your vagina. Truth is, you're guaranteed to have them for a long, long time, or at least until your vaginal mucosa resumes its prior level of elasticity, which is a feat that you'll come close to but never quite attain.

Strange as it sounds, this new talent that you have acquired can occur as a result of labial and vaginal edema caused by engorgement of the labia, or as a result of weight gain that occurs around the hips and vaginal area. Another reason for this new onset of vaginal turbulence is the widening of the pubic bone, which is a late second-trimester and third-trimester event that puts more stress on the pelvic diaphragm.

This is why your physician may talk to you about Kegel exercises, which are exercises whereby you strengthen the pelvic floor by urinating and stopping the flow of urination—contracting the muscles surrounding your urethra. If you're good at this, you can do it remote from urination, like when you are watching TV or at a traffic light—even in a convertible. (However, if you haven't quite gotten the hang of it, avoid the convertible since other motorists may wonder why your head is bobbing up and down rhythmically.)

Can I exercise during pregnancy?

Having been a marathon runner and currently a distance runner, I'm very supportive of women who want to exercise in pregnancy. Once the word got out that I run marathons, a multitude of runners seem to have become my patients—that darned Internet! I really like runners as people, but when I have them as patients we tend to be too much alike, and sometimes our personalities tend to clash. They are usually too Type A. Certain restrictions will be put on an athlete if they have twins, a history of preterm labor, an incompetent cervix, or an abruption, which is a separation of the placenta, or a placenta previa, which is a placenta that is covering the opening of the womb.

If the patient is spotting throughout the first trimester, she is not to exercise. If she has toxemia, high blood pressure or anemia, she will also be asked to avoid strenuous exercise. Toward the end of pregnancy, if she had a history of rapid delivery or advanced cervical dilation, I would also ask her to avoid exercise.

However, the benefits of exercise far exceed the risks. It will help you sleep and have a better sense of well-being, it will enable you to process and utilize your oxygen more efficiently, and it will help you avoid hemorrhoids and fluid retention. I firmly believe, having dealt with numerous athletes in my practice, that being one facilitates delivery. Exercise builds endurance and enables most women to more successfully handle a lengthy labor. It aids in the control of blood sugar and enables you to burn calories more usefully and, therefore, eat some extra pasta. It also helps in regaining a better postpartum figure.

Some important things to remember when you exercise are to always stay cool. It's better to underdress than overdress. Drink plenty of water, and never become overheated because the blood will go to the skin and, therefore, away from the uterus. If you are an average runner, as I am, you probably run between 35 and 40 miles per week. I would encourage you to run 2-3 miles per day and no more while you're pregnant.

If you are a marathon runner, you won't listen to anything I say anyway, because you will just want to run. But remember that as you get further along with the pregnancy, your hips are starting to separate, which will put more stress and pressure on the pelvic diaphragm and, hence, strain on your lower back. Not to mention that if you go running with a half-full bladder, you may leave a pee pee trail along your path. Take it easy, especially in the third trimester. It's not important to run a marathon this year. Look to the future to follow your dream.

I highly recommend swimming for those of you who want to exercise but are not athletically inclined. Not only will it burn calories and build muscle strength, but you will be amazed at how buoyant you have now become due to your brand new "floats." Also, your center of gravity is off a little when you are pregnant. If you tend to be a klutz and non-athletic, the water is safer because it is hard to fall in the water. But be careful getting in and out of the pool. We don't need you slipping and breaking an ankle after taking my little advice.

I also recommend pregnancy exercise classes. Our hospital offers a well-woman exercise class for pregnancy. I like it because it enables you to see what exercises you can and can't do during pregnancy. There are certain stretching exercises that will support the back and make you less prone to low back discomfort. The patients like these classes since they're not alone in looking like a water buffalo in a tutu, and in fact they even feel comfortable enough to wear their leotards. What's underwear among friends?

There are certain exercises that should be avoided at all costs in the second trimester, when the uterus starts to come out of the pelvis and, therefore, is not supported as adequately by the bony structures that surround it: for example, horseback riding, water skiing, or diving into a pool. Scuba diving is a no-no since decompression sickness could occur, which can prove to be fatal to the fetus. Sprinting uses too much oxygen, and downhill skiing can prove to be fatal to even the best skiers—remember poor Sonny Bono and Michael Kennedy. Also, jumping rope and hula-hooping may prove impossible!

No matter how graceful you may find yourself when you are not pregnant, your new shape has changed your center of gravity to the point where you may find yourself bumping into walls and falling quite easily. Riding a bike can also prove to be dangerous for you and hazardous to the pavement, since the chance of falling is quite high. Low back discomfort can also be pronounced.

Tennis and racquetball should be avoided in that they are high velocity, low impact sports with a lot of start and stop action that can cause the uterus to swing in the abdomen and can, as a result, cause a separation of the placenta. For the same reason softball should be avoided after you have reached the second trimester, but if you insist on playing, be sure to never slide to home base.

I have vaginal discharge; is this normal?

Leukorrhea, which can be a thin, milky, mildly sweet-smelling discharge, is quite normal. It may become progressively heavier throughout the pregnancy. Never use tampons in that this can be an access for bad bacteria to find its way to the cervix. If, however, the discharge is yellow, green, thick, cheesy, itchy or causes a burning sensation, in addition to having a foul smell, alert your physician. This can be a potentially problematic vaginal infection and/or a sexually transmitted disease.

I dye my hair and/or get perms frequently. What can I do?

Your best option is to shape your hair in an easy-to-manage style or put it up more frequently. Although some people are lucky enough to have a new luster to their hair, most of us are not as fortunate. Because of hormonal changes, permanents don't usually take as well as when we're not pregnant. You might find that the bounce you once had with a "non-pregnant permanent" makes you look more like you just stuck your hand in an electric socket when you are pregnant. No more Don King look-alikes, please.

In my opinion, avoidance is the best policy. The teratogenic (a drug-related malformation) potential of dyes and permanents has not been determined. Even though there is a good amount of chemical absorption through the scalp, it is very hard to measure birth defects using these chemicals. Avoidance in the first trimester is best. Then color and perm to your heart's content.

If I massage my perineum, will I need an episiotomy?

What I tell the patients is that whether or not you need an episiotomy depends upon the degree of elasticity of your skin at the time of delivery. It is also dependent upon the size and presentation of the baby's head, the length of labor, and the amount of swelling. However, if you want to start massaging your perineum in the early first trimester with olive oil, it certainly can't hurt. Now that you have an engorgement of your labia, it might even trigger an orgasmic response, so if it does nothing else, it may put a smile on your face.

What can I take for my cold symptoms?

Most of us when pregnant have a sluggish immune system, which can be compromised from the stress that pregnancy puts on our bodies. Most of us also feel run-down and tired, making us more prone to frequent colds. God in his infinite wisdom knew that modern medicine would have accelerated to the point where multiple medications would be available to diminish the symptoms of the common cold, among other things. For that reason He devised a mechanism known as the blood barrier.

The placenta is a wonderful organ that allows very few drugs to pass through its interwoven capillary network. When and if a drug does pass through, the amount that is transported to the baby is minimized greatly. Therefore, many drugs can be taken in pregnancy without any complication to the baby. Many of the over-the-counter remedies can be used, such as Co-Tylenol, Sudafed and Robitussin. Of course, if the symptoms do not subside, you should consult a physician. Most antibiotics can be used in pregnancy; very few cannot. Tetracycline derivatives are contraindicated, as are Floxin and Cipro, which can affect bone development of the fetus. For questions about medications and their possible adverse effects, I refer you to www.otispregnancy.org/hm.

I have a hot tub or a sauna. Can I go in it when I'm pregnant?

Basically, you don't want to raise your body temperature over 102° F for more than a ten-minute period of time. Most of us are incapable of doing that without melting, even in extremely hot baths or hot tubs, unless, of course, you're related to Richard Pryor. The first trimester is really the time period that you want to avoid this exposure since it can result in birth defects or developmental problems with the baby's spine and nervous system. Believe me, most women will spontaneously get out of the hot tub when the heat becomes too unbearable. If you live in the desert or have no pain receptors in your fingers or toes, remember to get out of your hot tub in ten minutes.

NINE MONTHS TO GO

TO TEST OR NOT TO TEST— THAT IS MY QUESTION

Here we go again. Even though I know I explained this a few pages back, you are still wondering if testing is for you. I can't give you the answer to that question. I can tell you all the reasons why testing is recommended and what tests are recommended at what times. And even though we did that already, let me reiterate now that you have had some time to digest what I already have said.

If you are over the age of 35, at the first prenatal visit your physician should discuss with you the value of genetic counseling and testing. Each patient has a completely different belief system. Some couples are so excited that they are pregnant, they very often don't wish any intervention to be done and are willing to accept whatever God grants them. Some couples are fearful of finding out bad news and would rather enjoy their pregnancy without the knowledge of having a child with a chromosomal anomaly. While the risk of chromosomal malformation does rise every year after the age of 35, with a 1 in 270 chance of Down syndrome at 35, it is ultimately your decision what precautions, if any, you wish to take. Please remember that younger women can and do give birth to babies with Down Syndrome. Until recently, testing has often been overlooked in this population.

Before you can make a decision, it is important to know the difference between a screen and a diagnostic test. A screen measures the chemicals in the woman's blood and combines the results with the woman's age and with ultrasound testing of the fetus. A screen does not diagnose a chromosomal abnormality, but rather it estimates the risk of having one.

A prenatal diagnostic test is either an amniocentesis or chorionic villus sampling. It is invasive and should be considered by women of any age at increased risk of having a child with chromosomal abnormalities. The diagnostic testing is offered if a woman had a prior baby with a chromosomal abnormality or has a fetus with a known structural abnormality (e.g., a heart defect or spinal abnormality), or if she or the father of the baby has a chromosomal abnormality themselves.

The advantages of first trimester screening include

1) Knowing as early as possible if the baby is affected.

2) Greater privacy in decision-making at a time when others may not be aware of the pregnancy.

3) More time for decision-making and preparation for having a child with an abnormality.

4) If the couple would consider terminating, the procedure is more widely available and safer if done before 14 weeks of pregnancy.

Some women do not want to have a screening test of any type. It is important to discuss those wishes with your practitioner. The choice to pursue testing is highly individual. A woman may choose not to have a first trimester or integrated screen for the following reasons:

1) If her prenatal care begins after the first trimester, she will no longer have the option for a first trimester evaluation. If so, she will still be offered a second trimester ultrasound and a quad screen, but she may decline. Once she is in the second trimester, termination is no longer an option and the patient may therefore not find the need to get tested at that late juncture.

2) The test may not be available in local or extremely remote areas.

3) Intervention and diagnostic testing such as a CVS (chorionic villus sampling) may not be available at her location.

If I do have genetic counseling and don't want to do anything about it, what good is it for me to have it?

My response oftentimes is that it could prove to be reassuring. A woman whose tests show an increased risk of Down syndrome can choose to have further testing to determine if the baby is affected. If the woman chooses not to have further testing, the infant may be tested after birth.

Genetic counseling can help parents balance the risks, limitations, and benefits of prenatal screening and diagnostic testing. Talking with a counselor can help the parents identify the issues that are involved in terminating a pregnancy and of raising a child with Down syndrome. In any event, when a child does have a handicap, such as a heart defect, then arrangements can be made for that child to be delivered at an institution where cardiac surgery can be performed right after delivery if necessary, which would avoid some of the emotional trauma of having to transfer your baby without you.

By the same token, this knowledge can prepare the parents for the inevitable. Certain chromosomal abnormalities are incompatible with life, and if a person's baby is going to have this genetic condition, she may not wish to continue the pregnancy but rather to terminate it and get on with her life and attempt another pregnancy. Career-oriented women realize that it is difficult enough to raise a healthy, normal child as opposed to one with a multitude of handicaps. For this reason, they may also wish to undergo genetic evaluation.

So tell me again, what test should I get? Did you say I should get a CVS?

No, I didn't say you should get a CVS. Yes, a CVS will give you a 100% assessment of your child's chromosomal status, but you are not a candidate for it unless you are over 35 or have had an abnormal first trimester screen or a significant family or personal history.

As a way of expounding on the genetic abnormality issue, the topic of CVS, or chorionic villus sampling, should be brought up with your physician if you have any questions or if you desire to have it done. Because of the availability of excellent screening tests, insurance will not cover the CVS if you just want to have it done regardless of your candidacy. If need be, these procedures can be done by a high-risk pregnancy doctor. If the tests are offered to you for one of the reasons above, but you are unsure as to how to proceed, a genetic counselor can meet with you and give you the statistics as to your risks of having a child with an abnormality vs. the risk of loss from having the procedure done. If the procedure is done in expert hands, the likelihood of a problem is quite low. Generally the CVS is done pending a discussion of the first trimester sequential screen.

The CVS can be done by either cervical or abdominal approach, in which a small catheter is placed into the cervix and a piece of the placenta is removed and sent to a genetic lab for confirmation of chromosomes. Depending upon the location of the placenta, the gestational age and the latitude of your uterus (anterior displaced or the degree of retroflexion), the perinatologist, who also does an ultrasound, may elect to proceed with an abdominal procedure as opposed to a cervical one.

Having had the CVS done both ways, I can tell you that for me the abdominal approach was easier, but that was because I had had prior surgery on my cervix, which can make dilation of the cervix and passage of the catheter more difficult. Having had surgery would also play a role in deciding which method is best for you. The perinatologist may also make the assessment based on whether or not you have had any sexually transmitted diseases, cervical incompetence or prior abdominal surgery.

If the CVS is done abdominally, a small needle will be placed in the abdomen just above the pubic bone and a small piece of placenta will be removed. It sounds painful to have a needle in your abdomen, but as I mentioned to you earlier, I am the biggest wimp I know, and yet this was much less traumatic for me than having blood drawn. The only part that was uncomfortable was when the perinatologist had to jiggle the needle to remove the piece of placenta. I saw stars and wanted desperately to spit in his face, but the discomfort was luckily short lived, and I was able to reserve the opportunity to embarrass myself until much later in my pregnancy.

The advantage of having a CVS over an amniocentesis is that your results are obtained more quickly, before you actually feel fetal movement and experience the more pronounced signs of pregnancy; hence, if a termination needs to be performed, it can be done by means of a surgical procedure without your having to undergo an early induction of labor.

An amniocentesis is done later on, and although the results can be given now within 7-10 days, you are further along, anywhere from 15-20 weeks, when the pregnancy is not as easily terminated. Having had a late amniocentesis for lung maturity with my second pregnancy, I can tell you with all honesty that this procedure does not hurt nearly as much as the CVS, but its disadvantage is that the results are obtained at a much later gestational age.

If you choose not to have any means of intervention, most obstetricians will respect that decision as long as you are well informed of your risks. It is important to keep in mind, however, that even with a positive screen, if you choose to assess your baby's well-being without knowing the genetic complement while pregnant, there are some non-interventional ways to assess the pregnancy. For example, a Level II ultrasound can be done by the perinatologist, during which he more accurately assesses the fetal anatomy to assure the absence of chromosomal abnormalities and rules out the potential for other defects that can prove to be devastating at the birth of your child if you are not prepared.

The doctor's looking at the fetus with a more upscale ultrasound unit, in addition to his advanced level of training, can assure us with almost 90% accuracy that there are not any fetal anomalies present. If there is any uncertainty, however, based on his findings, then you have the option to proceed further with an amniocentesis if you so choose. You must keep in mind, however, that there are very rare chromosomal abnormalities that are very subtle and cannot be detected by ultrasound evaluation. These are known as translocations. Although outwardly the fetus may not have any physical signs of this chromosomal abnormality, it may have growth or developmental problems or mental retardation, as well as other genetic problems that cannot be detected by means of ultrasound. This is why genetic counseling may be prudent in your decision-making process.

Many patients combine the Level II ultrasound with a quad screen. This was the standard of care up until 2008, when the first-trimester screen became standard because of people's desire to know more information sooner. If you present late for your care, the quad screen and ultrasound may be your only option for neonatal assessment.

The quad screen involves taking one tube of blood from the mother that enables us to determine the fetus's risk of chromosomal problems. This test, done between 15-20 weeks, combines the pregnancy hormone HCG with estriol and with a fetal protein which is excreted by the developing fetus (alpha fetal protein). An excess amount can imply neural tube defects (defects in the spinal cord or nervous system development). A decrease can suggest Down syndrome or other such related chromosomal disorders.

There are very few false negatives with the test, but a large number of false positives due to its over-sensitive nature. There are more false positives with this means of assessment than there are with the first-trimester screen, which is also why the second trimester assessment tool is falling by the wayside. Although I warn patients ahead of time of the false positive potential, some wish not to have testing done because of the undue amount of anxiety that it could cause them. Again, what option is right for you will be mutually determined by you and your doctor at your first prenatal visit.

You have now survived your first prenatal visit. You asked your questions, you are informed of how the pregnancy will proceed, you have met the office staff and the nurses, and you got along well with Mr. Scale. You were even able to pour the urine from the cup to the test tube without getting it all over your hands. Additionally, you have developed a rapport with your physician, and therefore it is now guaranteed that you will feel more comfortable, confident and in control than when you walked into the office earlier. On the way out the hairy lady didn't look so scary, and the burper was smiling. So go home, get some rest, buy some broccoli, put your feet up and drink your milk. It's time to go on to the first trimester.

Books for a Down Syndrome Pregnancy:

A Parents' Guide to Down Syndrome: Toward a Brighter Future, by Siegfried M. Pueschel, MD. Paul H. Brookes Publishing Company, 2001.

Babies with Down Syndrome: A New Parent Guide, 2nd edition, by Karen Stray-Gunderson. Woodbine House, 1995.

Gifts: Mothers Reflect on How Children with Down Syndrome Enrich Their Lives. Edited by Kathryn Lynard Soper. Woodbine House, 2007.

Gifts, Vol. II will be available in 2010.

Websites for a Down Syndrome Pregnancy:

National Down Syndrome Congress and National Down Syndrome Society:
http://www.ndsccenter.org

Dr. Leshin's web site for Down Syndrome health issues:
http://www. ds-health.com

Joann Richichi

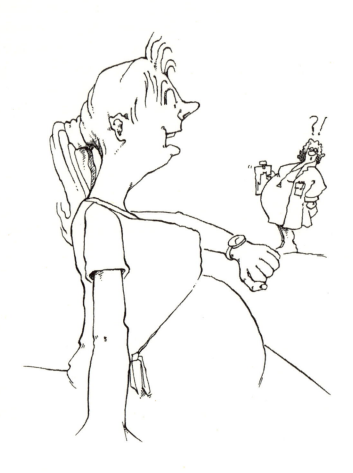

So Doc, who's due first?

Chapter 4

It Happened One Night

Now you know you are pregnant. There just ain't no doubt about it. There is no turning back. You went for you first prenatal visit. You heard the heartbeat. Even though it sounded like the pounding hoofs of a running racehorse, it was indeed your baby's heart. You did in fact get pregnant on that night you thought you only rehearsed.

You're as nauseous as can be and your breasts are so tender you wish you could just pop 'em. You've got the bloat. You look and feel fat. You are weepy because you don't feel pretty. You're irritable because nothing seems to fit. PMS was a walk in the park compared to this. You're sleep-deprived from worry, and anxious from fear. But don't fret. These mood swings and bouts of weepiness, feelings of fear mixed with elation and indifference, are all part of the first trimester. And the first trimester is already almost over.

As you approach the second trimester, you will feel a renewed sense of calmness, and your family members, whom you have now told after your first prenatal visit, will feel much less compelled to send you on a free, all-expense paid trip to Alaska for the remainder of your pregnancy. Just think, by the time you have left the office after your first prenatal visit, you are actually well into the first trimester—week 10 of 12. Not that your bizarre behavior is any reason why we don't wish to see you any sooner!

You may not want to tell any friends or relatives until your doctor actually confirms in big print, "Yes, you are pregnant!" Afterwards these friends will undoubtedly tell you they knew it—you had that "glow" about you. "What glow?" you ask. "Are they talking about that greenish-yellow glow after I leave the ladies' room each morning?"

Around this time your body will begin to feel different as well—fuller, more uplifted, happy. You're downright bubbly. You can't hold it in or you will bust—and to your surprise, you do now have one, as many an unsuspecting eye may have noticed.

I will divide the trimester chapters into four basic sections:

1) What you are to expect or feel during each trimester

2) Commonly asked questions and concerns

3) Problems that can arise in each trimester

4) When to contact your practitioner

Most important and pertinent questions do get answered in the first prenatal visit. Most patients have already accumulated their armamentarium. If you are a career-oriented neurotic or an intellectual piranha, you would have come to that visit very well prepared. Having already been pregnant for ten weeks, you would have probably read every book published on pregnancy.

It is in the last two weeks of the first trimester that most patients are going to pull that horrid paper out of the back pocket of their jeans as I'm slowly trying to make my exit. Still, I am often fooled by the freehand sign. The patient talks to me—nothing is in her hands, she's laughing happily, and all of a sudden she leans forward, and I know it's over, especially if her paper is crinkled.

As she opens the paper she says, "Oh, just one more thing, doc"—then I know for sure I'm in trouble. It is at this time that the loony-tunes and the career-oriented neurotics are going to ask the majority of their questions. Don't you worry, that is what we docs are there for. Please be kind and keep the list down to one page, as much more than that can cause a rapid increase of gastric enzymes in your busy physician's esophagus, which will in turn cause him to use up the patient samples of Mylanta.

The most common thing that most women experience in this trimester is nausea. It usually begins about two weeks after the missed period. Contrary to popular belief, it doesn't occur only in the morning; for most patients it is an all-day affair. It is at this time your bathroom may prove to be a safe place. It is also at this time in your life that the bathroom floor will be the cleanest, since in between bouts of vomiting, you may feel compelled to clean around the base of your newfound friend. No more toilet dust bunnies in your house.

Another common experience is uterine cramping. This can be a totally normal sensation in the first trimester, when women complain of mild, menstrual-like cramps. I reassure them by explaining that the uterus is a muscle, and as it grows it will cramp. Severe pain, however, is a different issue that we will talk about later and should always be brought to the attention of your practitioner.

Fatigue can be very common at this point, and your level of activity can be somewhat diminished. First-time moms often have concerns about their ability to be a mother, and they tend to get anxious about the baby's health. Career-oriented neurotics are most alarmed by fatigue because of their concerns about being able to work. Cool your jets, ladies. That pregnant body of yours is now working harder than ever before, and once you adjust to the emotional and physical demands, you will be right back in the saddle again.

It is prudent to get as much rest as possible and pamper yourself. Remember that fatigue can be made worse by too much rest; therefore, don't become a couch potato. Instead, go take a hike. Walking can lessen the degree of fatigue. I also stress to my patients that they should sleep often, eat well, exercise frequently and take 50 mg of vitamin B6 daily.

Frequent urination occurs due to the increased body fluids that are now present, the increased efficiency of your kidneys, and the fact that the pregnant uterus is now pressing on the bladder and will do so up until the fourth month, after which time the kid's bony little head will come right down against your bladder and cause a whole new pressure sensation. It is not uncommon for pregnant women to have episodes of enuresis (bedwetting). Don't be embarrassed. Just limit your fluids before bedtime, play Hawaiian music and buy your partner a float.

Just about every patient type experiences constipation except for the perfect priss. She doesn't get it because she is eating the perfect amount of fruits, vegetables and grains. She is increasing her fluid intake and she is exercising 2-3 times weekly, which will not only decrease the constipation, but also the flatulence. The perfect priss will never fart, gulp or gorge. She will always be a perfect lady. You know her—she is Bree on *Desperate Housewives*, and her tiny bouts of uncontrolled flatus might smell like the early-morning rose of springtime. Or maybe we smell the small tube of disinfectant spray she commonly keeps in her purse so that she can act above and beyond the other members of her species.

Palpitations are common towards the end of the first trimester. They may occur as a result of increased blood volume, which can make the heart need to pump more quickly to compensate. This can make you quite anxious, and although it should be an infrequent occurrence, if it happens to you frequently you should notify your practitioner.

Sweating often increases in the first trimester and remains at an increased level throughout the pregnancy. Don't go to work without applying deodorant, or you may get fired, and justifiably so.

Excessive salivation is an unpleasant, yet harmless and common complaint in the first trimester. While looking like a mad, rabid dog at the dinner table may prove alarming to other members of your family, it really is of no harm to you or your baby. It is usually gone by the second trimester and is easily taken care of by using a minty toothpaste, rinsing frequently with salt water, and going to the high school playground, where you can compete in the long-distance spitting contest and undoubtedly win!

The career-oriented neurotics tend to be those who suffer most from gas and flatulence. These tend to be the women who are most stressed out with life in general. They also are working hard and, therefore, may often eat fast food instead of the more healthy fruits and vegetables that are recommended. If you suffer from gas, steer clear of the gas producers such as onions, cabbage, broccoli, sprouts and fried foods, and of course, those naughty beans. Never bend at the waist, unless of course what's behind you is a campfire whose kindling is dwindling.

You may have the pleasure of experiencing varicosities, or increased venous engorgement. No, that is not a map on your chest, and your partner will not find a buried treasure no matter how hard he looks, but rather it is the bluish coloration of the increased number of veins located underneath your skin. They tend to be much more vivid in light-skinned women.

I had one patient who told me that she went to bed one night and woke up with different breasts—they weren't her own. To emphasize her distress, she opened her blouse and said, "Look, doc, these are not mine." Strange as that sounds, this woman was quite serious. I sincerely had to convince her that she was not a victim of the booby snatchers.

You may experience breast change, sensitivity and discoloration. The sweat glands around the areola or nipple of your breasts may become raised and can resemble large goose bumps. Your breasts and nipples may darken, and they may engorge and become excruciatingly tender to the touch. As it turned out, my ex-husband truly enjoyed fondling my pregnant breasts. I recall one night when he tried to do so. I was irritable and tired, and my tolerance for pain on that particular evening was quite low. Although his gesture was quite sweet, I responded with the vehemence of a wild boar by saying, "Watch it, buddy. These babies explode on impact!"

In terms of skin changes, remember that glow we talked about earlier? It can be real due to the increased oils in your skin caused by the raging hormones. It is best to avoid makeup and keep your skin well cleansed so that your face will not resemble the glow of the full moon, as you may develop craters from having pustule eruptions. Most women do not get acne while pregnant. If you choose to see a dermatologist, tell him that you are pregnant, as some drugs, such as Acutane and Retin A, should *not* be used during pregnancy.

Now for the commonly asked questions.

I have a lot of discharge and I smell different down there. Can my husband have oral sex with me?

Leukorrhea of pregnancy does have a different, "sweeter" smell. The increase in the thickness and consistency of the mucous is very common, provided there is no itching, burning or foul smell. Oral sex is very safe in pregnancy. Remember, however, that the mucous is thicker, so don't tickle your partner while he is busy since any sudden inhalation can cause aspiration and choking and even death. This in turn can lead to a very unrewarding experience.

What kind of sports can I participate in?

As I mentioned earlier, some high velocity, low impact sports can be done in the early first trimester. The uterus at this time is still protected by the bony structures of the pelvis. After that time, however, sports such as racquetball, tennis and volleyball should be avoided, as should horseback riding, scuba diving, sprinting, jumping rope and hula-hooping. And please don't bungee dive whatever you do. Remember, any other non-contact sport in moderation tends to be okay, provided you keep cool and stay well hydrated. Consider spending half the time on your workout than you did in the pre-pregnancy era. Oh, and absolutely no skydiving.

Can I lift weights?

What I tell a patient she can lift is dependent upon what she had lifted prior to the pregnancy. One of my patients was a competitive weight lifter on national TV. She looked a lot like Lou Ferrigno as *The Hulk*, now played by Ed Norton, only she did not have green skin and she was a little shorter than he, but boy, was she scary-looking. There was no way I was going to tell that great big mamma to only lift the 10-15 pounds that I tell the average mother-to-be. She was a perfect example of how every patient is a unique individual and, therefore, the answer to every question should be tailored accordingly.

Will my breasts be the same after pregnancy?

No, honey. Just like in Cinderella, when the time is up things will be as they once were. Look on the bright side: Cinderella didn't lose her prince. I must tell you that this question saddens me. It is at times like this that I wish I didn't have to be so honest. Your watermelons will turn back to apricots. The only difference is that they will then look like the dried variety, for most of us, that is.

Will my breasts be the same with my second pregnancy as they were with my first?

My answer to this is also no. They will be half the size they once were. But it is better to have had bazungas at one time than to have never had them at all.

I didn't gain enough weight in the first trimester. Is that going to hurt the baby?

No, it won't hurt the baby, and some patients even lose weight thanks to morning sickness. A perfect example of how nature takes care of itself is that the fetus doesn't need increased caloric intake at this point since it gains body mass at a much slower rate than it does in the second and third trimester. However, now that you are twelve weeks, you want to try to gain at least one pound per week from weeks 12-36.

I gained too much weight in the first trimester. Now what?

The percentage of the baby's growth in the second trimester is based on the pre-pregnancy weight and the weight gain in the first trimester. However, it is important that you don't lose weight, but rather gain at a steady rate. It is also important now that you monitor more carefully the type of calories that you are taking in. It is the quality, not the quantity of food that needs to be emphasized.

When will we be able to hear the baby's heartbeat?

The average time that we begin to hear the heartbeat is 10-12 weeks. However, in some women who are exceptionally thin and have a very antiflexed, meaning forward displaced, uterus, fetal heart tones can be heard at 8-9 weeks, but this is not the norm.

I can't sleep. What can I take?

At this point, your mind may be racing. You should try to unwind after a long day. Get some fresh air. Try to have a light bedtime snack. Don't go to bed too early. Clear your mind with yoga and read a good book. Not sleeping will not hurt the baby; however, you may find yourself becoming more irritable due to lack of sleep. The old wives tale of drinking warm milk can actually help in that it can release the chemical serotonin, which helps you sleep.

Massaging the acupuncture points in the back of the head where the bony structure meets the neck, known as the occipital prominence, can also be helpful. Pillows that put point pressure on these areas are recommended in pregnancy, or you can do what I did, which is put two tennis balls in a sock and tie it at the end. The balls sit nicely as you rest your head. It also works to relieve tension that can build up in the back of the neck and shoulders. And remember, if you get frustrated, you can always throw them or use them to play fetch with your dog.

Chamomile tea is also safe in pregnancy and has natural herbal ingredients that can enhance sleep. I would drink cozy chamomile each night a half hour before bed. I don't know how well it made me sleep, but I do know it increased the number of times I went pee pee in the middle of the night. Benadryl is also safe in pregnancy. I don't recommend its use every night. But if you find that your lack of sleep is turning you into Cujo, I suggest you try an over-the-counter 25 mg supplement.

I get headaches often when I'm not pregnant. Will they be worse during pregnancy?

Occasionally they will be worse in the second trimester. In the first trimester they can be as a result of stress, tension or sinusitis. Get fresh air and drink plenty of fluids, and it is okay to take Tylenol and Extra Strength Tylenol as needed. Remember to ask your practitioner if he agrees with this. Some chronic migraine sufferers actually get fewer headaches during pregnancy. Others tend to get many more. Obviously, if you know what brings on an attack, try to avoid that culprit. A dark room, fresh air, and easy listening music can all help the headache retreat. If things get progressively worse, however, you should call your practitioner.

My mom and grandmother had terrible varicosities, which got worse when they were pregnant. Will I develop them?

Heredity plays a very important role in the development of varicosities. Hormones relax the venous tissue, and the increased blood volume results in their dilation. The hereditary potential of having faulty valves in the veins that do not aid in the flow of blood back to the body and away from the extremities can make these varicosities much worse. Prevention can help diminish them.

If you think you have the potential to develop them, don't gain too much weight, try to avoid standing for prolonged periods, elevate your legs when possible, don't strain with bowel movements, never bend at the waist, and don't wear restrictive clothing, since bands around the abdomen can make pelvic varicosities worse and cause discomfort. Varicosities will not harm the baby; however, it can make you uncomfortable in that your leg cramps may be worse and your tendency to develop superficial thrombophlebitis (clotting in the superficial veins of the leg) may increase. There are stockings that are recommended to be put on when you get out of bed in the morning and taken off when you go to bed in the evening. These stockings, called TED or JOBST stockings, are available at most pharmacies. The JOBST stockings will require a prescription, so discuss their value with your obstetrician.

I burp all the time. Will this hurt my baby?

The reason for burping more during pregnancy is that food moves more slowly through your GI tract. Therefore, bloating and indigestion are quite common. No matter how loud that burp may be, the baby is blissful and protected in its bubble of amniotic fluid. If anything, the gurgling sounds of your stomach and the pounding of your heartbeat are reassuring and comforting sounds that are mimicked for babies who have difficulty sleeping after their birth. For my own children, I bought a tape called, "Hurricanes, Tornadoes and Other Wind Storms." If you want to diminish the resonance of your burps for other family members, eat small meals, eat slowly, never gulp your food, avoid hot and spicy meals, don't smoke, and eat with your head up at least at a 30 degree angle. Antacids are safe; Tums or Mylanta before bedtime can diminish some of the gastric acids that may accumulate and cause esophageal discomfort in the morning.

I get nauseous and constipated with my vitamins. What can I do?

Building tolerance by ingesting vitamins before pregnancy and in the early trimesters can avoid nausea and constipation later on. Vitamins are encouraged during this time period for many reasons, one of which is that they can help prevent neural tube defects such as spina bifida (a failure of the neural tube to close in its development). Switching the preparation or taking the vitamin in the evening or after meals may diminish some of these concerns. Also, adding ginger tea may help you tolerate the pill. Or try supplementing with vitamin B6 temporarily until the nausea goes away.

Keep in mind that rather than have the patient take nothing, as sometimes is the case for those intolerant to switching to or adding different formulas (the wimpy whiners and career oriented neurotics), I tell them to just take two Flintstones vitamins until this nauseous time passes, which is usually the beginning of the second trimester.

If the large prenatal vitamin pills look like they should be consumed by a horse, cow or elephant instead of a human, fear not, for there are liquid formulas available.

I can't drink milk. Is my baby going to get enough calcium?

It is calcium, not milk that your baby needs, and calcium is found in numerous foods, such as hard cheeses, yogurt, green vegetables and almonds. There is also lactose-free milk or lactose-reduced milk. Those who cannot tolerate milk often become flatulent as a result of lacking the enzyme to break down components. There are Lactaid tablets available to promote proper digestion. I can't tell you how many patients discover that they are lactose intolerant when they are pregnant. They find an overwhelming need to drink milk despite the fact that it disagrees with them terribly. It is only after numerous episodes of diarrhea, bloating and farting that they finally succumb to the fact that they shouldn't drink milk —and this, mind you, is often the intellectual piranha.

I am a vegetarian with no meat in my diet. What can I do?

Not being a "beefeater" can be okay and still render a happy and healthy baby. Fish and poultry are very high in protein and lower in fat. Some types of vegetarians eat eggs and milk, which provide an adequate supply of nutrients to their diet. The strict vegetarians, however, need additional vegetables, beans and legumes to meet their requirements. Their diet should be high in pure soybean products to aid in the proper amount of calcium. Those vegans probably could own their own hot air balloon service and do quite well by not having to pay the expense for fuel.

By the end of the twelfth week, your fetus is about three inches long and weighs 1/2 ounce. Vasculatory and urinary systems are now developing, and its reproductive organs are complete. The second trimester will prove to be much more comfortable.

Problems that can develop in the first trimester:

1) *Ectopic pregnancy.* These occur in 1 out of 100 pregnancies on the average. People who are at risk for them are those who have had a previous ectopic pregnancy, PID (pelvic inflammatory disease, an inflammation of the fallopian tubes and ovaries), or multiple abdominal surgeries. If you have had a tubal ligation and feel that you are pregnant or have missed a period, you too can be at risk for an ectopic pregnancy. Having an IUD and conceiving can also put you at risk, as can exposure to DES (Diethylstilbestrol), which is a hormone that women were given in the '50s to prevent miscarriage.

The symptoms of ectopic pregnancy are usually brownish discharge with occasional nausea, vomiting and pain, which is usually in the left or right lower quadrant of your abdomen. If the tube is ruptured or leaking, dizziness and shoulder pain may be present. Any bleeding or pain in the first trimester requires investigation and possible intervention, and your physician must be notified.

2) *Miscarriage.* Nearly 10-15% of all pregnancies end in miscarriage, and 20% of these pregnancies end before the diagnosis of pregnancy is ever made. The symptoms may be a brownish discharge or bleeding, which can be heavy at times—soaking several pads in an hour. The pain is often a crampy discomfort. There are different types of miscarriage. An incomplete happens when some, but not all of the tissue is passed, so that patient may need a surgical procedure known as a D&E (dilation and evacuation of the remaining uterine contents). A threatened AB means that the pregnancy is threatening to pass but hasn't quite done so yet. A complete miscarriage means that all the tissue has passed. The uterus should stop bleeding over a relatively short time period, so a D&E need not be performed.

A missed AB may not be found initially because the patient may not experience any cramping, pain or bleeding; however, the patient may have had prior pregnancy symptoms which have quickly dissipated. With a missed abortion, on evaluation in the physician's office, fetal heart tones may not be heard or the uterine size may prove to be smaller than it should be by the dates given. Remember, if you are experiencing any cramping with bleeding, you must contact your physician, who will then make the appropriate diagnosis and management strategy.

Depending on the circumstances, there are times when the physician may give the patient the opportunity to pass the products of conception on her own. If she opts to do this, she will have bleeding like a heavy period for several days, followed by light spotting for several weeks to follow. There are some patients who do not opt for this since they would do better emotionally to end this very painful experience quickly with surgery. Others choose to avoid surgery if at all possible.

On an even sadder note, there are rare times that anomalies or teratogenic exposure may be incompatible with quality of life for the fetus. Or there may be times when a woman can no longer continue her pregnancy for mental, emotional or personal reasons. Once a woman has reached 13 weeks gestation, a generalist will no longer offer a termination, but depending on the circumstances, a high-risk pregnancy doctor might. If you elected to have a termination, you would probably not be reading this book. But if you do desire to terminate your pregnancy, there are many places you can go to have your needs met. Never seek this or any option without medical supervision and counseling.

3) *Nausea/hyperemesis.* This can occur in the first trimester and end by the 14th gestational week. The symptoms can be quite pronounced, including profound nausea and vomiting, inability to tolerate fluids, and a need for hospital admission with IV nutrition

and vitamin therapy. It rarely gets this serious and most times can be managed on an outpatient basis.

4) *Twins*. Although a twin pregnancy is considered high-risk, it does not usually present problems in the first trimester. Twins are usually diagnosed at this point in time because the uterus is larger than it should be judging by the FDLMP (first day of last menstrual period) date given by the patient. The physician will order an ultrasound, which will confirm twins. There two different types of twins, identical and non-identical. There are no precursors to having identical twins; this is one egg that happens to split early in gestation. Non-identical twins can occur as a result of fertility drugs or in-vitro fertilization, or can be of hereditary potential based on the maternal side of the family. It occurs in 2 out of 100 pregnancies.

The average caloric intake with twins should be 300 more calories daily than for a single pregnancy for a weight gain of approximately 35 pounds. We will talk further about twins as we talk about the third trimester, because twins put you at increased risk for preterm labor, high blood pressure, edema, varicosities, gestational diabetes, and a potential C-section. Aren't they lovely?

Most patients breathe a sigh of relief when they overcome the concerns of the first trimester. After this point in time they no longer worry about the potential for miscarriage. It is also when the nausea diminishes. It is the second trimester when most patients feel at their best. So let's look forward to it as we discover this trimester together in Chapter 5.

Chapter 5

Happy Days Are Here Again

Well, ladies, you've made it through to the best time of your pregnancy—the second trimester. This is when your anxieties are at their lowest. You no longer have the fear of miscarriage, and you're not quite thinking about labor and raising a child. This is a time of cruising and snoozing. Although your energy level will be at its highest, when you do rest and sleep you will do so in a much more fulfilling manner.

Bloodwork will be obtained only once in this trimester. That will be between weeks 15 and 20 and will include the triple screen (if you opted for a CVS instead of a sequential first trimester screen) or a quad screen if you either chose not to be tested in the first trimester or couldn't be tested because of presenting late (after week 13-14) for your first prenatal visit. An ultrasound will be done in this trimester as well in order to assess dates and fetal development. With the ultrasound, a good anatomical survey will be done so that if you desire to know the sex of your baby, you can ask at that time.

My anxieties and my problems were most pronounced in my third trimester. However, I had several in the second trimester—shopping for a bra at this time became a frightening experience. As I'm sure you have gathered from reading this book thus far, the Lord was kind enough to grant me many talents and abilities. In the process He did, however, forget a couple of body parts which suddenly showed up during the late first and early second trimes-

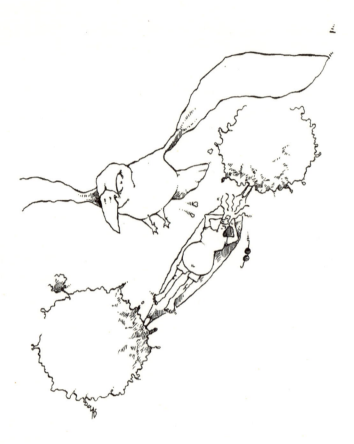

ter. Therefore, I no longer had the luxury of lounging around in my T-shirts and tank tops—I actually needed a bra!

As you may soon find out, pregnancy bras are about three times the size of an average bra. They have multiple clamps to account for the expanding breast and abdomen. They are heavier and have more elastic in the hopes of offering more support, and the straps are very wide. Wearing this made me feel like Houdini in the Chamber of Doom. Therefore, I reserved wearing them for the third trimester. I then purchased nursing bras instead of pregnancy bras since they offered support and the peek-a-boo windows for nursing when the time came. When you are pregnant in the hotter months, they can be a good source of ventilation. For the second trimester I settled into a normal Playtex Cross Your Heart fitted (bigger cup than I'd ever had) bra and was quite content.

The second major anxiety occurred on the evening of my high school reunion. Having not seen these people for over fifteen years, I was anxious to begin with. Although I had on a miracle bra and a low-cut dress, I couldn't even enjoy the cleavage that I had for the first time in my entire life because I was also dealing with the fact that my rear was keeping pace with my growing abdomen. Therefore, my fellow classmates looked at me with wonder and awe. Did she just get fat or is she pregnant? There was no mistaking the inquisitive look that I saw in the eyes of my ex-boyfriends. There was no fooling me—they were thinking, "She finally got implants! I'll be darned."

My third major anxiety was when I told my fellow residents that I was pregnant. Not one of them seemed happy for me. I was crushed. But I came to realize that, to them and other fellow workers, pregnancy meant lack of productivity. They wanted to be sure I admitted just as many patients as they did and took as much call as they did. Let's face it, nobody wants to work extra if they don't have to. My expanding abdomen was to them a sign that those overworked and tired residents might just have to work harder.

So I, being the wonder woman I thought I was, worked my ass off. (No I didn't, because no matter how hard I worked my ass was still there, and so was my belly.) Because I was trying to prove myself, I worked myself right into preterm labor. This meant that I would not only have my scheduled maternity leave, but an additional leave to prevent the preterm labor from worsening. Boy oh boy, did they hate me. I later tried to make it up to them by coming back and doing only night call. That gave them the chance to sleep each and every night for a month and a half. They still were not overwhelmingly thrilled with me. As I said, I was hurt by it, but I got over it.

What I wanted to tell my fellow residents—and everyone else, for that matter—is that pregnancy is not easy. And it is very, very hard to work a demanding schedule and maintain pregnancy comfortably. Jeez, we are doing a service to God and humanity by being pregnant. We are saving the human race and allowing it to not become extinct, which it would if man himself had to bear its fruits. We should be praised and thanked by all the non-pregnant folk who are discriminating about our current state of being!

You will be discriminated against at work. It is a known fact. Not all will look at you with a raised eyebrow and bitter smirk of discontent, but some will. You should be prepared for it and not stressed out by it. If it doesn't happen and you think I am a lying fool, great! I am really happy for you. That happens sometimes. But you must understand, having been subjected to the "smirk" by a room full of fellow residents who were learning the art of bringing life into our world, I am skeptical that your fellow workers will truly be happy for you.

If you think you are being treated unfairly at work, please don't sit there and take it. Talk to someone you can trust, like your supervisor or someone from the human resources department. Review your employee handbook so you know your rights. If you feel your job is too stressful for this and other reasons, try to hang in there. If you leave you will have to deal with a new set of stresses, like how to handle a new job you will soon need to leave. Your potential employer has no right to ask you if you are pregnant (unless, of course, you already look like a cow). He can't deny you a job if he discovers your secret, but let's face it, he may. If he gives you the job (before you start to show) and then you ask about your maternity leave, he will never trust you or like you again. There goes your opportunity to advance up the ladder of success. Every job stress and circumstance is different. If it is getting to you, let your practitioner know.

Now is a good time to mention environmental hazards. Although this was not a source of anxiety for me, it may be to you. If you know the substances that you work with, you can call the toll free pregnancy hotline (1-888-722-2903), or you can look on the Internet for their teratogenic potential (capability to produce a mal-

NINE MONTHS TO GO

formation in development). If your job does expose you to hazards, ask to be transferred. Maybe it is a good time to get away from that stuff anyway.

Whatever your job description, trust me, it just got harder. There are some things you can do to make it easier:

1) Take a load off whenever you can and elevate those poor dogs.

2) Stretch when you can. I don't care if you look like a fat monkey.

3) Get some back support if you job requires lots of sitting.

4) Empty your bladder when you have to. Don't be ashamed to go pee-pee. If your employer gives you a hard time with this, wet his chair. And for that matter, every chair and couch in the place. Believe me, if anyone has that much urine in her, it's you.

5) Lift carefully and only if you have to. Don't bend over at the waist—bend your knees.

6) Meditate and breathe deeply whenever possible. Like when your boss is in your face with a list of things you have to do NOW.

7) Do what your body needs to do when it needs it. Listen to your inner voice. That is, if you can hear it with all that rumbling going on.

8) Dress comfortably. Don't wear anything restraining. Don't wear high heels if you don't have to.

Bottom line is, don't let work get to you. Just be happy for this special time in your life. Nothing else is as important right now as you!

One less traumatic anxiety is shopping for clothes. At this point in your pregnancy you most likely will be too small for maternity clothes and too big for your old clothes. It was at this time that I got excellent use out of my scrubs. They were roomy and I felt like I was in PJ's all day long.

Doing surgery with my fellow attendings became a little anxiety-producing for me. Surgery, which I normally loved, became a particularly exhausting burden. During my first pregnancy I was a resident. As my abdomen protruded, it became more and more difficult for me to get close to the surgical table. It was also easier for the attending to elbow my breasts or abdomen, which during a long case was so painful that I desperately wanted to get even and squeeze his testicles. I restrained myself, realizing he had to grade my operating ability as a resident.

In my second pregnancy, I was the attending, and allowing my male residents to perform the vaginal surgeries under my direction proved more embarrassing to them than it did to me. It was funny seeing how confused and uncertain they became when they realized that both of us couldn't fit in the small area between the patient's legs.

However, for the most part, the second trimester was my favorite time during pregnancy. It was after this point when the hassles of preterm labor overcame me. For many of you this will be a happy and fun time devoid of stress, accompanied by a minimum of flatulence and bloating, occasional headaches, and a definite increase in your appetite.

Food aversions and cravings may be common at this time. They don't have to be worrisome, but they can be weird. Recently, a patient of mine in her 23rd week was at the front desk making an appointment when I noticed her munching on something that appeared somewhat odd. When she left the office, my receptionist noticed that she had left a piece of her munchies—lo and behold, it was a dog biscuit! I kid you not! It was then that I truly understood what my patients meant when they stated they had a ferocious appetite while pregnant.

NINE MONTHS TO GO

It is at this point that leg cramps may be present, although less severely than in the third trimester, and you may notice some mild varicosities and venous engorgement. Your abdomen may become itchy from dry, scaly skin. It is also now that you may develop a lower abdominal ache secondary to the stretching of the ligaments, or an increase in Braxton-Hicks contractions. Your constipation may increase as a result of the slowing of the gastrointestinal tract motility and the pressure of the expanding uterus on your colon, which may also cause your hemorrhoids to resemble a budding rose in springtime as it comes into full bloom. Fear not, there are ways to dull their hue, as we will discuss shortly.

For the most part, your time in the office will be much quicker than it was in the first or will be in the third trimester. The nurse will weigh you and check your blood pressure and urine as she normally does. However, your visits with the doctor will only include a quick palpation of your abdomen, a measurement of the size of your uterus, and a listen to your baby's heart. You will be asked whether or not you have any questions, and if you don't, you're out the door—wham, bam, thank you ma'am. The career-oriented neurotics like the brevity of these visits since they are anxious to return to work. Things also tend to go smoothly for the intellectual piranhas. They may even become frustrated in that there are a limited number of questions that they may find themselves asking.

The wimpy whiners and loony tunes feel lost and lonely and are often found hanging out talking to the receptionists or spending an exorbitant amount of time in the waiting room bathroom. Ironically, the perfect priss may require comforting. She will want to be reassured that she is doing everything correctly. At this point, she may become somewhat sensitive about the change in her abdomen, the loss of her once petite waistline, the growth of her thunder thighs and the loss of her ankles. This apprehension can sometimes turn to anger, as it did on the night of my high school reunion—not that I'm a perfect priss by any stretch of the imagination. At one point during that evening I came very close to pulling the microphone out of the hands of the band leader and yelling, "These suckers are real, damn it! They're not implants, and I'm not fat, I'm pregnant!"

It is at this time that you may wish to take a family member to the office to listen to the baby's heartbeat, even your other children. Most of us, especially mothers like myself, understand the need to bring siblings along for doctor visits. Therefore, in my office we have an area where siblings can color in the event that the mom needs to be examined or has a multitude of questions that need answering.

On several occasions, however, I have been in awe of how many patients wish to have their children in the exam room while they are being examined. I'll tell you the story of Mrs. Green, for example. Mrs. Green was in to have her 36 week culture, which requires an internal exam. It was summertime and she didn't have a baby-sitter. Her sons were four and six years old. When I told her that it was time for her internal exam and culture and asked her if she would like the boys to go out and color, she insisted that they should remain and she would hold their hands while I examined her. In case you've never had the pleasure of bringing young children with you into the examination room, you have never fully realized how curious they can be—especially boys.

So picture Mrs. Green holding on to these two children as they're pulling and tugging her arms as I am examining her and placing the speculum in its proper location. Finally, she let go of the children and I had two little assistants at my side. I looked at my assistants and they looked at me, and one of them asked with pure innocence, "What's hiding in that hole, doc?" Before I could answer the other child said, "It's dark in there!"

Well, the moral of the story is, unless you want your youngens to see where the sun never shines on their mama, you really should keep them out of the exam room while you're being examined. As you can see, that is where Mrs. Green got her fictitious name. She was an intellectual piranha who believed in teaching and educating the children. While I honor her idealism and her honesty, in my opinion the definition and multi-capabilities of the vagina would be better as a self-taught educational experience that Junior can acquire later in life. Those two little boys will have plenty of time to discover their own cave of dreams—why does it have to be their poor mama who shows them the way? I mean, life is short, but it ain't that short.

Most patients bring their significant other to their second trimester visits. However, if you've had a bad month of being mean to your partner, or of eating too much junk food or smoking too many cigarettes, you might want to leave your partner at home for the visit. Trust me, no matter how much he loves you, he will rat you out. Go ahead, try it if you don't believe me.

Now then, shall we continue where we left off? It is in this trimester that you may find yourself in denial as you try to fit into your once-appealing wardrobe. Remember, bigger is better. Looking like a tent is far more rewarding than having your underwear show from splits in your pants. Be comfortable. So what if maternity clothes are expensive and ugly? You'll need very few items, as it's only a few months, and you may even choose to borrow from friends and family.

Also, a word of caution: Beware of the pregnant panty. They are not only ugly but extremely uncomfortable; therefore, as I have learned from my patients, a nice bikini style, cotton, three sizes bigger than normal, is much more appealing and comfortable. If, however, you happen to have purchased your underwear prior to reading this word of caution, you may decide to take them with you on your next trip to Switzerland or France, in that they will serve as an excellent parachute if the need should arise.

One word of reassurance is that if you are fortunate enough to be less endowed, such as myself, it is at this point that you will feel absolutely no jealousy toward the buxom bunch that you have known in the past. They are the ones who look miserable, their faces drawn and tired from carrying that extra load they must keep in that horrible pregnancy bra. You, on the other hand, are still in your Victoria's Secret bra and panties, feeling footloose and fancy free.

FREQUENTLY ASKED QUESTIONS

I'm experiencing numbness and tingling in my hands. Is this normal?

My answer is yes. You're probably experiencing carpal tunnel syndrome, which is caused by the fluid that has accumulated in the fingers and around the ligaments in the wrist. Try to avoid sleeping on your hand; wear wrist splints, which are available in most drug stores; take some vitamin B6; and take in some natural diuretics, such as vegetables. You may want to steam the vegetables and drink the water—this is high in diuretic potential as well as nutrients and vitamins. Also, drink plenty of water, and avoid anti-inflammatories, which work very well for the swelling, but cannot be taken during pregnancy.

The numbness will be made worse if there is excessive use of your hands. I suffered from bilateral carpal tunnel with both pregnancies because of the surgery that I was doing, which involved a lot of bending at the wrist. If you are a typist or work on the computer, you may suffer from this discomfort. Artists who paint and draw frequently may be burdened with this as well. Keep in mind that it may last up to three months post delivery.

Don't worry, you will soon be able to give your partner the finger without it feeling all numb and tingly. If it persists, you should talk to your primary doctor, who may refer you to an orthopedic specialist. Most of the time it will go away, but if you are prone to it, it might return with a vengeance when you are older, like it did in my case, even though I am not truly older.

Can I continue my cocaine habit?

Now what do you think? No… And before you ask, you shouldn't continue smoking either. Not only are you putting yourself at risk, but you are potentially causing harm to your developing fetus. Sorry to sound so abrupt, but it can only cause harm, so why do it? Smoking cigarettes is not nearly as bad a habit as cocaine, but if you can stop, please do.

Can I use my cell phone?

Yes, except while driving.

Can I use my microwave?

You'd better, because I know you are going to be way too tired for stove top cooking by the time you get home from work.

Should I wear a seat belt?

Yes indeed. If your belly seems to protrude too much, which it is more likely in the third trimester, just put the abdominal strap below the belly. It is much safer for the baby to endure the pressure of the strap then the abrupt injury it might sustain in the case of an accident. Babies are floating and cushioned by lots of amniotic fluid, so please don't worry about the pressure of the strap. To avoid injury from the air bag, sit as far back as possible while driving and all the way back as a passenger.

Sometimes I feel a lot of movement and other times none at all. Is my baby okay?

Around 16 weeks you will begin feeling some type of movement, and it will become more pronounced between 24 and 28 weeks, when the baby is most active. At this point you and your partner can not only feel it move, but you may see it as well. After the 28th week the kicking will be better perceived as a more definitive and direct movement. Yes, this is when he starts to show his love.

It is not uncommon to feel a limited amount of movement in the early second trimester. It is a time when the baby's nervous system is immature and, therefore, the baby's sleep cycle is longer. You may notice that the movement is dependent upon your level of activity. Very often, a very busy day may be accompanied by a decreased perception of movement. On a very quiet day you may observe an increased degree of movement, when in actuality the amount is quite the same; it is just your perception that is different.

My legs cramp at night. Is this normal?

This question is most often asked by the career-oriented neurotics who work long hours and are on their feet the whole day. They also have a tendency to wear high heels, which exaggerates the extension of their calf muscles and causes cramping later on in the evening. The wimpy whiner does the absolute worst with leg cramps and may even cry about the distress it is causing her.

Having had these cramps, I know they can be quite intense. Let's face it, after a long day your legs are tired from carrying the extra pounds. The swelling is also compressing your poor little tired blood vessels. Leg cramps can also be caused by a decrease in calcium and potassium and an increase in phosphorus Some women feel compelled to drink a lot of milk because Aunt Matilda told them to. But actually, while milk is great for your bones, it may increase the amount of phosphorus in your bloodstream. Therefore, substitute with alternative sources of calcium, and be sure to take your vitamins.

Additionally, try performing exercises before you sleep in which you stretch the calf muscle by leaning against the wall and repeatedly elevating your calf by bending your knee and flexing your foot. If it is too late and you are lying in bed when the cramps strike, flex your ankle and point your whole foot slowly up and then slowly down. Do this on both sides several times before going back to sleep.

If you have a bad cramp, your leg may be tender the next day. They usually occur in the middle of the night while you're sleeping. Be prepared for them. Don't do what I did, which was to punch my husband in the chest in an immediate signal for him to rub my calf. (Remember, I am currently divorced.) You are probably young and naive and want to prevent that from happening to you. So, rather than wreck your marriage at this juncture, straighten your leg and extend your foot. This maneuver will stretch the muscle in spasm and diminish the pain.

Sometimes warm compresses on the lower extremities may also help. If you have a waterbed, turning up the heat may be ideal, for you anyway. If, however, you have continued pain in your extremities with redness or swelling, be sure to notify your doctor.

I stand all day. Is this safe for my baby?

It most certainly is. Despite what you may have learned as a child, women were not meant to stay on all fours. Therefore, Mother Nature had to compensate for our ability to stand erect. While there is plenty of support to the pelvic diaphragm, prolonged standing can cause additional swelling and an increase in the varicosities. Therefore, try to elevate your legs whenever possible. If rest periods are difficult to achieve, support stockings may become necessary and can prove to be quite helpful. Even though you may not be able to obtain disability at this point in your pregnancy, cutting your hours may be a good idea. Talk to your employer about leg elevation and rest periods. If he proves to be an unreasonable prick, then ask for a doctor's note, or call me and I will get my cousin Vinny to take care of things for you.

I'm such a klutz lately. What's wrong with me?

This becomes a particular problem for the intellectual piranha because she, too, may occasionally become ditzy and forgetful like the rest of the pregnant population. This may also heighten her degree of clumsiness. The increase in hormones during pregnancy results in elasticity of the joints and an increase in their mobility. I had one patient who fell down the stairs almost ten times while pregnant. She was constantly getting monitored for having fallen. Obviously, she was no gymnast. I cautioned her that if the fall was severe enough, and she hit her abdomen hard enough, it could cause the placenta to separate, known as placenta abruption.

Finally, despite my insistence that she stop her unnecessary household work of going up and down stairs, she fell while carrying a laundry basket and broke her ankle. Although she was quite upset, and naturally so, I told her that broken ankle was the best thing that could ever have happened to her baby. Needless to say, it certainly diminished my concerns and fears for the safety of that child's intra-uterine environment.

Patients in their second trimester begin to retain more fluid, which can cause a decreased perception of the grasp that is necessary to lift and move objects. At this point, using your antique fine crystal is a definite no-no. This pregnancy-induced carpal tunnel syndrome may cause you to break and drop everything you touch.

Your center of gravity has also shifted due to your expanding abdomen and the increased extension of the muscles in the lower back, making it easy for you to topple over. I got a phone call once on a hot summer Sunday afternoon from a patient who was a 30-week-pregnant perfect priss. She was out buying watermelons for her family barbeque. While bending over the bin to find the perfect melon, she toppled over and could not get out of the bin on her own. She was lifted out by some attendants in the Shop-Rite while other consumers stood and watched in horror and sheer amazement. Having had this accident, she wanted to know what she should now do. I told her to go buy some blueberries; they were in season and much safer to reach.

Be careful while bending forward so you don't become the next watermelon lady. Exert extra caution while going up and down stairs, and use an elevator whenever possible. If you are a gymnast, the forward roll and cartwheel may prove to be exceptionally easy at this point in time. I would recommend, however, that you refrain from such high velocity activity.

Some patients, particularly the loony tunes, wimpy whiners and perfect prisses, will begin to wonder about pain management in labor. The wimpy whiners are starting to get apprehensive about the pain. The loony tunes are beginning to think about everything that might go wrong. The perfect priss just wants to make sure she is going to do a good job and not embarrass herself and, therefore, she may be very inquisitive during the late second trimester. The intellectual piranha will want to know the percentage of medication that will cross the placenta and how it may affect the baby. In general, I tell my patients that it is very good to anticipate what lies ahead and it's very important to be realistic and open-minded, because if you do so, you will not be disappointed. Of course, I too, was a bona fide wimp. I firmly agree with aggressive pain management in labor, but I give the patient the right to choose.

Should I take birthing classes, or will it be a waste of time?

For repeat moms who have had the experience recently, I feel that it would not benefit them very much. However, for first-time moms I believe that taking the classes can decrease anxiety, improve their ability to tolerate pain and teach them how to relax and use the necessary muscles in labor. Not to mention, they give the patient the opportunity during break time to vent with other expectant moms, which if done under the guidance of the instructor, should avoid mass hysteria.

I always thought it would be a good idea to incorporate singing lessons into the birthing classes, so that if you find yourself suddenly hysterical and unable to remember the relaxation techniques, you could always sing to relax. Although the sound of your voice may be gratifying to you, it might prove devastating to your very embarrassed partner. Birthing classes often allow you to develop a better rapport with your coach or partner. This will aid in lessening the degree of obscene gesturing and vulgar profanities that you might otherwise elicit in labor. The psychological instruction the patients receive during these classes will also aid them in using their pain in a productive fashion. Therefore, their partners are less likely to get punched and the obstetrician less likely to be kicked, bitten or scratched.

Of course, birthing classes aren't for everyone. Sometimes people choose to know very little because it makes them less anxious. Also, those that take the classes don't push any better or deliver their babies any faster or easier than those who don't. It's important to know your personality and your expectations, which will help your caregiver in determining if the classes are right for you.

Keep in mind that most obstetricians and the nursing staff will guide and teach you during your labor and delivery. You're not expected to know how to push, so they will work with you. Also, there are numerous tapes available in video stores which can instruct you on how to breathe and how to control your pain throughout labor. I highly recommend at the very least you review one of these tapes with your partner so you have an idea what to expect.

What can I do about these hemorrhoids?

Megarrhoids often show their angry heads during the second trimester. This is a result of the constipation from the prenatal vitamins with the added complement of the heavy uterus weighing down on the poor, crushed colon. Avoid constipation, sleep on your side, don't strain while moving your bowels, do Kegel exercises, use warm sitz baths followed by witch hazel soaks, and take Metamucil, which is a bulk forming agent and can aid in bowel motility. If things get out of hand, let your practitioner know so that he can recommend stool softeners and/or topical ointments. Avoid hot and spicy foods, and don't listen to the song "C'mon Baby, Light My Fire."

My abdomen is itchy all the time. What can I do?

Don't scratch! Aside from looking like an ape in the zoo, it will also cause excessive irritation due to the sensitive nature of your skin at this time. You can use lotions such as calamine or vitamin E-based creams. If a rash develops or if you notice itching all over your body, be sure to make your caregiver aware of this. There are certain pregnancy-related rashes that show up in the late second trimester and early third trimester.

NINE MONTHS TO GO

If I don't wear a bra, will I cause any harm?

I might ask, "To whom, you or your partner?" Although I poo-pooed pregnancy bras because of my own fear and apprehension, you may not have the luxury of avoiding them. They can prove to be quite useful in that they will give you more support and cause less pulling and strain on the pectoral muscles and breast tissue and, therefore, less tenderness. Not wearing a bra can cause a stimulation of the nipples, which can cause increased contractions or preterm labor. Also, it can cause the let-down and expression of milk.

Many women in the late second and early third trimester need to sleep with a bra, as they do once they deliver and are breastfeeding. This not only gives the added support needed, but also prevents milk expression into their partner's eyes while rolling over. While there are evenings when this might prove appealing when you have some built-up anger toward your partner, use caution. Remember who has the piece of anatomy that could wipe you out and put your wimpy little squirt to shame.

Can I eat fish? How much? How about sushi?

Fish and shellfish are an important part of a healthy diet. They contain high quality protein and other essential nutrients. They are low in saturated fat and high in omega-3 fatty acids (remember them?). A well-balanced diet should include a variety of fish and shellfish, which can contribute to heart health and children's growth as well as brain development.

However, the old saying "too much of a good thing is bad" tends to apply in the fish department. All fish and shellfish contain traces of mercury. Mercury occurs naturally in the environment and can also be released into the air through industrial pollution. When it accumulates in streams and oceans, it is turned into methyl mercury. It is this type of mercury that can be harmful to your unborn baby and young children. An accumulation of methyl mercury has been linked to developmental delays and brain damage.

Fish absorb the methyl mercury as they feed, and it can build up in them over time. Some fish are more prone to the build-up than others. The larger the fish, the more likely it will have accumulated methyl mercury. Those fish that have lived longer have the highest levels simply because they have had more time to accumulate it. The fish that fall into this category are swordfish, shark, king mackerel and tilefish.

Canned chunk light tuna generally has a lower amount of mercury than other tuna. Believe it or not, fish sticks and fast food sandwiches are low in mercury, but I would not recommend them because of the extremely high fat content. You can safely eat two three-ounce cans of tuna per week in addition to having one 6-ounce fish meal at dinner. This is more than most Americans consume per week. If, however, you eat way more fish than this per week, keep in mind that, just like in fish, methyl mercury can build up in us, and it may take a year to clear from our systems.

You should eat no more than two fish meals per week, and you can eat up to 6 ounces in each meal. If one week you ate five meals of fish, don't worry. One week does not change the overall level of methyl mercury in the body, so just remember to cut back the next week.

If you like to fish and to eat what you catch, check your fishing regulation booklet for information about the recreationally caught fish in your area. You can also contact your local health department for information about local advisories. If you want more information about the levels in various types of fish, see the FDA food safety web site or the EPA fish advisory website.

Although I love lox (raw or smoked salmon), it should be avoided because it could be contaminated with listeria. Listeria is a bacterium that might also be found in imported soft cheeses, which is why they too should be avoided in pregnancy. Listeria has been found as the causative agent in some miscarriages. It is a bacteria that is known to cross the placenta and can therefore be a cause of preterm labor and neonatal infections. Although we were not talking whenever possible. If you're good at headstands, you may be asked to do this several times a day. The stitch is often cut at week 37 or with the confirmation of fetal lung maturity.

(4) *Placenta previa.* As mentioned earlier, this occurs when the placenta lies low, blocking the exit into the birth canal. It may be partial or complete and can result in excessive blood loss. It may be detected as a result of second trimester bleeding or seen in the second trimester ultrasound. Many times the placenta migrates toward the area of increased blood supply, which is in the fundus (top) of the uterus and, therefore, away from the opening of the cervix. On rare occasions, it completely covers the opening of the os (cervix), which can result in episodes of bleeding throughout the pregnancy as the uterus expands and contracts. At the time of delivery, if a complete or partial previa is detected, a C-section is performed. Depending on the degree and amount of bleeding episodes, the patient may be able to stay at home with strict bed rest, or she may need to be admitted to the hospital and on occasion may need to be delivered early.

(5) *Polyhydramnious.* One other condition that may be detected in the second trimester, either by ultrasound or by measuring the size of the abdomen and indirectly measuring fundal height (height of the pregnant uterus), is excessive fluid surrounding the baby. Increased fluid, often a third trimester event, can also be detected by a sudden increase in weight with the patient insisting she has not eaten more or did not feel as though she gained weight. Her legs may suddenly become swollen, and she may have developed diabetes. She may have Rh immunization disease, which can be a result of lack of prior immunization if Rh negative. She could also have an abnormal antibody that can have an effect on the fetus; however, she would have been screened for this in the initial prenatal visit, and this should have been anticipated early on in the pregnancy.

Polyhydramnious can also signify a problem with the fetal swallowing mechanism, which can be a result of a chromosomal abnormality. Therefore, an amniocentesis may need to be performed to rule out this possibility as well as to diminish the degree of fluid that is surrounding the baby. Polyhydramnious can be a totally idiopathic event, meaning no known cause, and can prove to be a totally benign event as well. Therefore, if you are found to have an excessive amount of fluid, don't become anxious. Allow your practitioner to do the proper workup necessary. Many of the occurrences I have just mentioned are quite rare.

(6) *Oligohydramnious:* This is decreased fluid around the baby. Oligohydramnious can sometimes suggest decreased development in the fetal kidneys or a leaking/ruptured bag of water that went otherwise undetected. This, of course, warrants further investigation.

(7) *Excessive snoring:* A less worrisome complication that may occur is due to edema and nasal congestion, coupled with the increased blood supply to the nasal area. While this complication may not prove devastating to you, it may cause rapid abandonment by your partner. I can't tell you how often a partner has asked me in a pleading fashion, "Doctor, will she ever stop snoring?" "Yes," I tell him with sympathy and understanding, knowing that this poor person has spent many an evening on a couch or recliner.

Well, girls, it's time for bigger and better things as we enter the third trimester! See you there.

Chapter 6

She's a Brick House

The Third Trimester

While you may think the Commodores were referring to you when they sang this song, in actuality they were not. You're now in the middle of your third trimester—33 weeks, to be exact. While you're sitting in the waiting room observing the different-sized abdomens, you suddenly realize that yours may very well be the biggest, and that now you're responsible for being the "team leader." All eyes are looking to you for support and encouragement.

You're irritable, however, due to the increasing episodes of constipation, the leaking of milk from your breasts, your aching hemorrhoids and your increasing episodes of shortness of breath. The evening before, you experienced a bout of nasal congestion, making it quite difficult for you to sleep. And to top it off, your husband said you sounded like a warthog in heat. The blackened circles around your eyes, of which you are self-conscious, make it hard for you to look into the eyes of your fellow pregos.

Just when you think you can render some support, a foot is suddenly jammed into your rib cage, causing you to let out a sigh and bend forward. Just as you do so, the head of your baby, which has not quite descended into your pelvis, bounces off the back wall of your bladder, causing a sudden surge of urine, which wets your new red slacks. You look around to see if anyone has noticed. You get up slowly, heading for the bathroom. You're pulling your blouse down to cover your wet spot just as someone walks out of the bathroom—an old friend, who is only 10 weeks pregnant, and she raises her hand to greet you.

As you raise your hand to greet her, the wet spot is now obvious to her and everyone else in the waiting room. The embarrassment causes a sudden rise in gastric acids, which turn your hello into a loud burp that sounds like a deep resonating noise that only a psychopath would make. "Hellooooooooow" you say as you cover your mouth in shame.

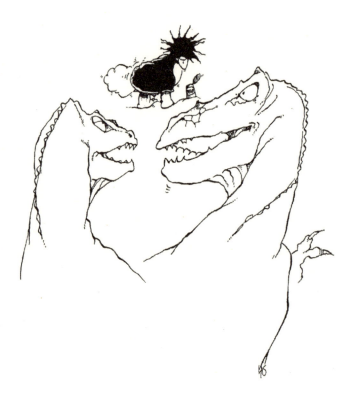

I think it is a pregnant human. I hear they can be fierce.

NINE MONTHS TO GO

Your bubbly friend looks at you frightened and confused. You don't seem at all like the person she once knew. It is now that you truly realize how eager you are for this pregnancy to be over. The calm, floaty-type feeling you experienced in the second trimester has come to a rapid halt. You have had enough!

When we think of the third trimester, we think of weeks 28-40 (37 if you're lucky, and 42 if you're not!). Therefore, it is a long time. And just the thought that it can be longer than the other trimesters is sickening. It's more like a tri and a half. It's harder than a triathalon. What do those athletes know anyway? They haven't done anything much if they've never been pregnant. You're on your way to a tripregalon, and that is much harder.

Many of the questions we reviewed in the second trimester will also be asked in the third trimester. If you are an intellectual piranha, you would have asked them well before this time. If you are a perfect priss, you may have thought about asking some of them but wouldn't have. After all, you could never admit you were in any way constipated. It is here that the wimpy whiners and loony-tunes truly declare themselves.

There is not much in the way of change from what we have already covered, other than you have the opportunity of drinking the sugary glucola, after which your practitioner will test your blood sugar to assess your risk of developing diabetes in pregnancy. For that reason, and because the third trimester is so long, we'll talk mostly of the things that occur in the middle of that trimester, weeks 30-36 until your actual date of delivery.

I tend to have a skewed negative view of this trimester because I spent weeks 25-33 and 34 respectively, on my back with complete bed rest. I really shouldn't complain; after all, I gave myself the opportunity to experience this portion of my pregnancies to the fullest. Every symptom and every concern was magnified since I had nothing more to do than think. As you can see from reading this book, thinking can prove to be a very frightening experience for someone like me. Nevertheless, being the physician that I am, I will try my best to render support as we go through this chapter together.

THINGS YOU MAY EXPERIENCE

You may notice an increased amount of constipation, heartburn and indigestion. The fetal movements will occur with more regularity and with greater vehemence than they did earlier on. You may occasionally experience headaches and episodes of dizziness. The headaches may actually prove to be less pronounced than they were in the second trimester. Because of the engorgement of your gums, you may notice bleeding around their edges. No, don't worry. You won't look like Hannibal Lecter in *Silence of the Lambs*, but after eating chips or tacos, exercise caution while smiling! Your leg cramps may become more pronounced due to the increased edema (swelling) in the lower extremities.

Low back pain will become a definite issue, especially for the career-oriented neurotics who are on their feet constantly. Superpubic (the area just above your pubic bone) and mid-pelvic pressure and discomfort will become an issue for the intellectual piranha who sits by the computer night and day. Sitting straight, although good for your posture, is not always good in pregnancy since it can increase the pressure on the upper thighs, where your abdomen has been sitting for the last 5 weeks, making your upper thighs and lower extremities as numb as cucumbers. This pressure enhances the swelling in the lower extremities. Your poor innocent little blood vessels are becoming compressed from the accentuated load.

If you can pull your computer keyboard out toward yourself as you type, you might have less lower extremity edema and pelvic pressure. Use a round pillow in your lower back region to support your lower back. Using a keyboard can also result in carpal-tunnel-induced pain and numbness in both hands. Using a wrist-rest while typing may prove comforting. Also, if carpel tunnel becomes an is-

NINE MONTHS TO GO

sue, you may need to limit your workload. Wrist guards can be worn to keep the wrist from flexing. The bending at the wrist can make the numbness much worse.

In addition to varicose veins and hemorrhoids, you may develop an itchy abdomen and will more than likely have difficulty sleeping as a result of this and other burdens. Braxton-Hicks contractions will become more prominent. You may become irritable from the annoying persistent cramping in your lower abdomen. The leaking of colostrum from your breasts will begin to occur in this trimester and may have already wet your new silk blouse in the trimester before. Coughing, laughing and sneezing may cause a leakage of urine and/or a constant trickling of urine. In other words, you won't need to be a comedienne at your next family outing to be known as a piss-a.

Emotionally, you may find yourself more eager to get things over with, and you may begin to feel apprehensive about the baby's health, the labor and the actual delivery. It is not uncommon, due to this anticipatory excitement, that you may experience some absent-mindedness. It is at this point where the career-oriented neurotic and the intellectual piranha may experience their first panic attack, since they now feel compelled to settle issues from childhood that they had nine months to do, but avoided. It is much easier to read a book about childbirth and management of your newborn than to think about how the experience will truly affect you.

As the 37th week begins to roll around (and that's not a pun on words!), it is now the perfect priss who is starting to feel anxious. Everyone wants pregnancy to end, ironically, except the perfect priss, who is now beginning to fear labor and delivery. Although she desperately wants her body back, she is worried ad nauseum about being a wimp and having a bowel movement in labor. Fear not—those buckets under the delivery tables serve more than one purpose.

It is around the 38th week that the wimpy whiners will begin to get anxious and apprehensive, for they are suddenly remembering how hard it was to put their last tampon in—what the hell will it feel like to push this bowling ball out of this tiny little hole? Not to mention the fact that someone showed them forceps in the birthing class, which they are now fixated on and begging their practitioner not to use under any circumstance. The intellectual piranha just saw *60 Minutes* and has a multitude of questions regarding the use of vacuum cups and the millimeters of pressure that are required to effectively extract the baby from the birth canal. We reassure them regarding the methods of vacuum and forceps application and the fact that there are certain times when these instruments are required.

These wimpy whiners also have many questions regarding the epidural and when they will be able to receive it. They are frightened by the size of the needle, however, and wonder if there is any way around that. You assure them, however, that by the time they are requesting that epidural, they would not care if the needle was the length of a flagpole! They'll just want it, and they'll get it.

It is in the third trimester that the laid-back, experienced type will remind the practitioner that they will not need an IV, nor will they require fetal monitoring while in labor. They would like a room with a Jacuzzi, and they will insist upon walking in early labor. The intellectual piranhas that have read everything there is to read regarding pain relief in labor will tell you that they may have their hypnotist present during labor and delivery. I always tell the patients that provided labor is moving along as anticipated, they can have whoever they wish to have in the room with them. Inevitably, it is the patient who will be kicking the hypnotist out as she demands her epidural. It is not the power of hypnotism that I am condemning, but rather the intensity of labor that I am emphasizing.

Overall, I do believe the third trimester is the most anxiety-producing for the career-oriented neurotic. She is the one who is most worried about being a "bad" mother. She is also the one who needs to constantly remind herself that she is woman, hear her roar! And she often will roar in her physician's face, especially about issues regarding the date of her delivery, induction or C-section, which she will feel compelled to schedule in advance.

I felt the urge to mention these categories in this trimester because it is the time period when we all seem to show our true colors, as we often become most of what we are under times of stress. Don't worry. Your practitioner knows what to expect from you and, hopefully, will also know how to reassure and comfort you during this very exciting yet anxiety-producing time of your pregnancy. Your practitioner may encourage you to formulate a birthing plan, so that he knows what your expectations are and what is going on in that active mind of yours. He will also be able to cue you in on how unrealistic your goals might be. In any event, writing things down can make you feel more in control and a little less neurotic.

Your physician will be checking you every other week from weeks 28-36, and every week thereafter until delivery. He will be listening to the fetal heartbeat, checking the height of the fundus (top of the uterus), and seeing if the size is proportionate to the estimated size of the fetus. This will enable him to determine if you will have a large for gestational age baby or a small for gestational age baby, or if there is too much or too little fluid surrounding the baby.

Depending on the size, he may or may not order **non-stress testing (NST)**, which is a test that assesses the baby's heart, similar to an EKG. It is the nature of that heart rate, its accelerations and decelerations which enable us to determine the baby's wellbeing in utero. He may or may not also recommend **biophysical profile testing**, which is an in-depth ultrasound and NST to assess how well the baby likes the intrauterine environment.

Such maternal conditions as high blood pressure, smoking, advanced maternal age, lupus, or other chronic medical illnesses are additional reasons to do such testing. He may order such testing if he is suspicious of an intrauterine event such as an abruption, diminished amniotic fluid, or an overabundance of fluid (oligohydramnious, polyhydramnious). He may do so if he suspects calcifications in the placenta or early aging of that placenta. He may recommend testing in the event of an IUGR (intrauterine growth restricted fetus).

Testing may also be recommended as a result of your increased perception of decreased fetal movements, resulting from the diminishing amniotic fluid after week 36. A certain degree of diminished activity after the 36th week can be totally normal, as a result of the decrease in amniotic fluid coupled by the increase in fetal size, but it can be an indicator of fetal compromise. He may ask you to monitor fetal movement counts on a regular basis. If you tend to feel less than six movements in the hour after eating a meal, your doctor may wish to be notified of this decrease, at which time testing will be recommended.

Testing is usually performed after the 32nd week, when the fetal neurological system is developed enough to assess the heart rate in relationship to viability and fetal compromise. An ultrasound may be ordered around week 36 to assess the estimated fetal weight of the baby. If it is over the 95th percentile, it may alert the practitioner to the potential of shoulder dystosia. We will discuss this potential malady when we talk more about labor and delivery.

In addition, the third trimester will include checks of the patient's urine for sugar, protein and infection. It is at this point when pre-eclampsia, or toxemia of pregnancy, may show its ugly face. The practitioner may also assess your reflexes to see if they are hyper, which can be an indication of pre-eclampsia. He will examine your hands and feet for swelling. Your weight and blood pressure will be checked weekly, because a sudden weight gain can mean an overabundance of edema, a sign that pre-eclampsia may be developing. This tends to be the time when most pregnant women, regardless of the category in which they find themselves, are united in making the same comment to their practitioner: "Oh, no, doctor, the ten-pound weight gain this month is not my fault. It's my swollen ankles, see?"

Remember, it is between the 27th and 29th week that the one-hour sugar study (glucola) will be done. This test will sometimes be done sooner if you are at risk for gestational diabetes, and will not be done if you are already a known diabetic whose sugar is monitored regularly or who is already on insulin. If you are not known to be diabetic, than you will be given a sugary drink and asked to remain available so that one hour later, your blood can be drawn to assess the possibility of glucose intolerance, that is, the inability of your body to assimilate all those cream puffs you ingested over the last several weeks.

People who are over the age of 35 are more likely to be prone to gestational diabetes, as are those individuals who have a strong family history of Type II (late onset) diabetes. People who gain an excessive amount of weight during the pregnancy can also be at risk for diabetes. People who are of American Indian decent or Eskimo decent are also at higher risk. If the test is positive (a number above 140), then a three-hour test will be ordered for you shortly thereafter. For that test, you will arrive in a fasting state and your blood will be drawn at hourly intervals. Gestational diabetes may mean that you will need a special diet to control the insulin regulation, which means, of course, you will have to avoid Mama's brownies. Or you may need to be placed on insulin.

In addition, if you are a smoker, or in the expanding group of patients who are over 35 years of age (AMA, or advanced maternal age), your practitioner will review the necessity of fetal heart rate testing or non-stress tests (NST) and/or biophysical profile. Remember too that age 45 is the new 35... So eventually this category of AMA will be of the older population, but for now you are still deemed advanced at age 35. But from my point of view you are still a baby.

At week 36 of your pregnancy, a vaginal culture will be performed. This is the beta strep culture to see if you are harboring this particular organism that is asymptomatic in most women but can prove to be harmful to an infant born to a mother who is carrying the bacterium. If you prove to be a positive carrier it can easily be treated in labor with IV antibiotics. If you should deliver before 36 weeks and a culture was not yet done, you will automatically be treated for beta strep, because the risk of neonatal infection in not treating a potential carrier is high. The 36 week check will also give your practitioner a chance to recheck your pelvis in relationship to the presenting fetal part, which is hopefully the head. This assessment will allow him to determine the likelihood of a successful vaginal birth.

Remember that "term" can be between 37 and 42 weeks. Practitioners in this day and age will not allow a woman to go beyond her 42nd week of pregnancy because the risks of fetal demise and compromise are much higher after that point in time. Between 40 and 42 weeks, an NST or biophysical profile and fluid volume checks will be done to assess fetal well-being. A diminished amount of fluid can imply that the fetus will be in danger of developing a cord entanglement or compression and, hence, fetal distress. It could imply a prematurely aged placenta, one that will no longer function appropriately. These are indications for delivery.

The physician will check your cervix frequently to assess the optimum time for delivery. Many patients have the luxury of delivering in the 37th or 38th week. Inductions of labor are oftentimes not done in this time period in that the practitioner is still concerned about the possibility of lung immaturity, unless a compromising neonatal complication arises or a maternal condition, such as pre-eclampsia, manifests and worsens. The benefits of delivery must be weighed against the potential risk of lung immaturity at birth. Therefore, in most instances inductions are done in the 39th or 40th week provided those complications do not supersede the need for fetal maturity.

Because of my overzealous desire to end my own pregnancies, I tend to be more liberal about performing inductions. Once I know that the cervix is favorable and the patient has reached her due date, then it's gone baby gone. However, if fetal testing is adequate and maternal conditions are well maintained, induction is by no means a necessity, but rather an opportunity to end your sentence.

If it is your first pregnancy, we tend to be less liberal with induction of labor because the risk of needing a C-section will be made much higher. The reason why the thinking gets somewhat foggy is that having a C-section is no longer the risk it once was. Many women opt for it as a preference, which we will talk more about later in this book, when we review mode of delivery in more detail.

All my partners, except the one that has had children, are much less liberal about offering induction of labor. They feel that a natural transition into full-blown labor will lessen the likelihood of needing a C-section, and they are right. They are also of the opinion that cervical change, if it occurs on its own, will be less uncomfortable than with a full-blown, aggressive induction of labor. Honestly, labor is labor, but induction makes it all happen so much sooner and faster, and how could that be bad?

While most practitioners feel early inductions can push one to the point of a prolonged labor and unnecessary C-section, I feel that once a patient's due date is reached, an induction is a fair alternative to being in a state of perpetual discomfort. That is, of course, if the right factors are met for induction, barring other potential needs for C-section. If you are 39-40 weeks and don't wish to go beyond your due date, talk with your practitioner to see if you are a candidate. Also, if you don't have a medical reason to be delivered sooner than the date your body chooses to go into labor, then even if you are offered an induction and meet all the criteria for a successful vaginal birth, you don't have to take the opportunity. Of course, if you are offered an induction and decide against it, I think you need your head examined instead of your vagina. We will talk more about this when we talk about labor and delivery.

From my experience, the career-oriented neurotics will tend to ask for induction most often because they are usually a Type A personality and on a very strict schedule. They are very concerned about when they can return to work. They are also the ones most focused on how effaced or dilated they are—that is, how thinned out or open their cervix is. Don't expect to ask a career woman who is 37 weeks pregnant or beyond how she is without hearing an answer like, "I'm okay—I'm 2 centimeters, 50% effaced and plus one station, how are you?"

Once the perfect priss reaches week 40 she, too, will request an induction, the reason being that it seems as though it has been an awfully long time since she went to the day spa out of fear of not being able to tie the robe appropriately. Her nails and hair are not looking quite as good as they should, and she has finally had enough. She just has to get this thing over with. So what if she poops when she's pushing? Such is life.

COMMONLY ASKED QUESTIONS

I'm afraid of losing control and having too much pain. What can I do to prepare myself?

Nothing! No one knows what labor feels like until it is experienced. Since I am the biggest wimp I know, I want to reassure you that I have devoted much of Chapters 7 and 8 to pain management in labor. I totally respect your fears and anxieties because I had them too. I am a firm believer that labor should be enjoyed and not endured, especially because of all the hell you have had to put up with for the last nine months. The birthing class will make you aware of your options, and your practitioner should review these options with you preceding and during delivery.

I want to experience labor naturally. Do you have a problem with that?

The answer to that question is no, I don't have a problem with that, but you may. I try to encourage all of my patients to keep an open mind. You may have an excellent tolerance for pain, but nothing short of the passage of a kidney stone is quite like the pain in labor. Although the outcome is far more rewarding than the passage of a crystalline rock, the discomfort, from what I am told, is as intense. Luckily I have never passed a kidney stone, but most of my patients who have think labor is a piece of cake. Therefore, if you haven't experienced the miraculous event of birth in the past, I caution you to not hope too much for that which you may not accomplish. I am very proud of my patients who do labor naturally, and if that be your wish, more power to you. However, please don't try to be a martyr. You've already endured enough.

I'm short of breath all the time. Is my baby getting enough oxygen, and will he have a lower IQ if I don't breathe properly?

Shortness of breath doesn't mean that either you or your baby is not getting the proper amount of oxygen. Many changes occur in your respiratory system during pregnancy. In the last trimester the expanding uterus presses against the diaphragm, making little room for the lungs to expand. Relief occurs when lightening occurs. (No, you will not be struck by a bolt from the sky. There is no easy way out of this.) "Lightening" is the descending of the fetus into the birth canal. In the first pregnancy, this usually happens at approximately 36 weeks. If this is your second or third pregnancy, it may happen later. Although shortness of breath is quite common, if it is severe and accompanied by rapid breathing, a blue discoloration of your lips and fingertips, and/or chest pain, you should call your doctor, and he may recommend an immediate trip to the ER.

I get pain in my rib cage when I take a deep breath. Should I be concerned?

The ribs undergo a flaring (a turning outward) to accommodate the expanding abdomen and to make room for deeper inhalation. This pain in the ribs from your brand-new pain in the ass can be quite intense, sharp at times, and can increase with movement and various position changes. You may take Tylenol or Extra Strength Tylenol and apply a warm compress to the back. On rare occasions, it may be prudent to see a chiropractor or a massage therapist, who can replace the rib to a less painful position. Let's face it, all of us could use an excuse for a good massage now and then. What better one than a rib that has popped out?

I am a moose. Will my baby be a cow?

As we discussed earlier, your weight gain in pregnancy does contribute somewhat to the size of the baby, as can gestational diabetes. It is with gestational diabetes that lipid deposits are more pronounced on the shoulders of the infant, making the baby look like a linebacker. This can make one more prone to a situation called shoulder dystosia, in which the shoulders get trapped in the pelvis after the baby's head presents itself on the perineum. We will talk about this in more depth when we get to the chapter dealing with labor and delivery.

If your weight gain is exorbitant, over 40-50 pounds, your physician may ask that you maintain a restrictive diet to prevent either gestational diabetes or a macrosomic (large for gestational age) infant. Remember, however, that genetics play a very important role as to the size of your baby. Very often I have seen obese moms deliver small infants. Therefore, to answer your question, you will more than likely not give birth to a cow, but I can't stress enough the proper management of weight control while pregnant to avoid other pregnancy-related complications. Just in case, perhaps you shouldn't name your baby Elsie.

My mom says I'm carrying low and very small. Does that mean I'll deliver early, and is my baby growing properly?

Remember, you will be told a multitude of things by various family members and friends. Some will make you worry. Try to put their advice and comments aside, because in many instances they will be misguiding. That is why your doctor will see you so frequently in the third trimester—to make sure that you don't listen to these people and to check if your size is appropriate. Carrying low does not mean an earlier delivery; it just means more pressure for a longer period of time.

NINE MONTHS TO GO

I'm carrying in the front, and everyone at my shower told me I am having a boy. Is that true?

Speculating on the size and position of a woman's abdomen is one of the things that most other women seem to wholeheartedly enjoy doing. However, there is no documentation in any medical literature to support these assessments. How you carry is dependent upon your size and shape and your height—whether you are thin, petite, heavy or voluptuous to begin with. It very often is not an indication of the size or gender of the baby you are carrying.

Believe me, I'm a very petite, non-voluptuous woman. By looking at me at 34 weeks, you would have thought I was delivering a full-grown buffalo. Yet I popped out a 4-pound, 7-ounce baby. Also, according to the wives' tale, if you're having a boy you carry in the front and maintain your prior beautiful facial features. If, on the other hand, you're having a girl, you tend to get bloated and gain a good amount of weight in your face, backside and legs. My mother-in-law, the dear that she was, told me that according to the old wives' tales, it looked like I might be having twin girls. In all honesty, my butt was very close to the size of Manhattan.

I can't tell you how many tall women present with this concern of carrying too small. If you're one of those women, you are very fortunate in that your pregnancy will show at a much later time, and your clothes will fit for a longer period of time. If you are tall, your torso is often elongated, so the growth in your uterus does not pose a threat to your diaphragm or pelvis as it does for a shorter woman. There is oftentimes less shifting in the pelvis to accommodate the baby, hence, less back pain. Medically, however, I have been unable to explain why much shorter women have a tendency to develop a bigger butt in pregnancy.

Since you are checking position, is the head down? Is the butt first or the head?

As part of the assessment of your pregnancy, your doctor will be checking for position. Especially in a first pregnancy, if the baby is breech, most practitioners would not want to deliver vaginally since they would be unsure as to what your pelvis is able to accommodate. Therefore, the assessment of presentation will become more important after the 34th week. It is by this point that the baby will find his positional niche. The overwhelming majority of infants become cephalic (head down) by that time.

If at 36 weeks in a first pregnancy the infant is still breech, the practitioner will talk to you about a procedure known as a version (turning of your baby from butt-first to head-first). He will discuss how this is done and if it is a feasible alternative to your having to have a C-section. We will go into more detail in our next chapter on labor and delivery.

Breeches are more common if a pregnancy is early in gestation, if the uterus is unusually shaped, or if there is an excess of amniotic fluid. Contrary to what your male counterparts have told you, it is not due to the baby having a large penis or very big testicles that are pulling the baby's butt down. It is also more common in a multiparous woman (a woman who has had more than one birth) and one in whom a prior pregnancy was breech as well.

While some physicians routinely perform C-sections for all breech presentations, believing it to be the safest route for the baby, many offer a vaginal birth with a breech in a multiparous situation. Several criteria must be met. The baby must not be macrosomic (must weigh less than 8 pounds). There should not be any evidence of placenta previa. The risk of prolapse of the umbilical cord must be minimal. It is preferable when allowing a woman to deliver vaginally that the presenting part be engaged into the pelvis when labor begins. It is also recommended that the fetal head is not extended, but rather that the chin be tucked into the chest and flexed. It is also recommended that the butt is presenting first, not one or two feet. The patient and everyone in the delivery suite should be ready for a C-section.

If you are 34-36 weeks and your practitioner finds that you are breech in your first pregnancy, there are several maneuvers that

NINE MONTHS TO GO

you can do to help turn the baby. One is the knee-chest position, in which you lean on your elbows and knees and bend forward. It is a good idea to ask your partner to rub your back while you are in this position to relieve some of your stress at the same time. This position is referred to as the doggie position, speaking of which, you should refrain from having any family pets in the room with you at this time. This position may aid in the turning of the infant while relieving your stress. Another tactic is swimming in a pool on a float while kicking and leaning forward on your abdomen. Another maneuver is riding the express elevator to the penthouse of a skyscraper. Last but not least, there is skydiving at a 30,000-foot altitude, but I do not recommend this to my patients as the risk/benefit ratio seems hardly worth it.

I'm afraid of dying in childbirth. Is that likely to happen?

With modern medicine, even if your pregnancy is the highest of high risk, you have more of a chance of dying on the way to a movie theater than you do during labor and delivery. Medicine may have its shortcomings, but managing labor is something we've learned how to do efficiently. Fewer than 1 in 11,000 women die in childbirth. This includes those women who have chronic heart conditions and serious illnesses, and those who give birth in shacks, bathrooms and taxi cabs with little to no medical assistance.

I'm 5 feet tall and very petite (although not so petite while pregnant). Will I have trouble delivering my baby? Will I need a C-section?

When I think of the answer to this question, I think of my Jewish boyfriend in medical school, who was a wonderful person and as cute as can be. I wasn't in love with him, but I did love him, and although he wanted to marry me, I found every reason why I shouldn't. He was short (you would think I was tall). He reminded me of a cute little boy that I wanted to cuddle with, but not marry. And I thought he had big lips. I should have paid more attention to his beautiful baby blue eyes, but I was young and naïve, and all I really cared about then was being a doctor.

Then one day, my mother squeezed my cheeks with such intensity that my dimples took on a new depth. She asked, "How could you be so stupid? It's not what's on the outside, it's what's on the inside, not to mention he has a lot of money. Besides, he's a wonderful person, and Jewish men make excellent husbands."

Fortunately, when it comes to giving birth, it really is what's on the inside and not the outside. For the most part, regardless of your size, it is the shape and size of your pelvis in relationship to the shape and size of your baby's head that is important. Women of Asian descent usually have a smaller pelvis, but luckily their infants are smaller as well. The potential for C-section may come into play when this Asian woman conceives the child of a 6'4" Norwegian linebacker. (You do remember it is Norway that is known for its whale blubber eaters and big babies.) When a doctor sees that couple walk through the door, he knows to sharpen his scalpels and prepare them for the inevitable.

I seem to be constantly leaking urine. What can I do?

For one thing, don't go visit Aunt Sally without bringing a towel to sit on. And above all, never sit on her brand new couch. The word will get out amongst the family members not to invite you over for holiday dinners. It would be no wonder if you get the metal folding chair when everyone else has a cushioned dining room chair!

You shouldn't limit your fluid intake. Hydration serves a very important purpose in the third trimester and should never be diminished. Remember to empty your bladder frequently. Bite your lip instead of laughing at everyone's jokes, do your Kegel exercises, and don't jump up and down at your baby shower no matter how excited you are about the 10th car seat that you have received.

I'm having twins. How will my pregnancy be different from everyone else's?

Well, at least you're not having octuplets, so consider yourself lucky! Honey, this question should have been answered a long time ago by your practitioner, and most likely was. You need your own book on twinning as well as your own personal psychologist for the postpartum period. I do realize that you may be suffering memory loss above and beyond that of a woman carrying a single gestation, and rightly so. You have a lot of concerns about the future, so I'll take a few moments to review some issues.

Before I go any further, I want to let you know that I am currently dealing with a close family friend who is now carrying her second set of twins! Could you imagine? Well, she couldn't either. The first set I could hold a little responsibility for, because I gave her medication to induce ovulation, which can increase the likelihood of twins. Her beautiful daughters, who are not identical, are currently three years old, and she is pregnant again with twins that she conceived all on her own. They are now in the process of finding a live-in nanny. Most of her concerns are about how life will be after the birth, not prior to it, and rightly so.

First of all, in order to answer this question as thoroughly as it needs to be answered, you need your whole Britannica series, but I'll try to limit it for convenience sake. Although many mothers of twins have normal, uncomplicated vaginal deliveries, the majority have the potential for many complications. In most cases, vaginal delivery of the first twin may occur without any complications. The second twin, however, may undergo an element of distress, necessitating an expedient delivery with vacuum, forceps or perhaps even a C-section. Both fetuses will be monitored throughout the whole labor. Once the bag of water is ruptured, one will be monitored internally and one externally. You must always be prepared to expect the unexpected.

Before you reach this time in labor and delivery, your pregnancy will be monitored closely with ultrasounds for growth of the fetuses. Very often a condition called discrepancy can develop in which one twin tends to grow better than the other. If this is the case, earlier delivery may become necessary.

You are more prone to hypertension, diabetes, pre-eclampsia, and excessive swelling. Bed rest may become necessary earlier on in the pregnancy, and preterm labor may be inevitable, necessitating a decrease in your activities and possibly medication to prevent the uterus from contracting prematurely. If both fetuses are breech, a C-section will become necessary in the 38th week. If the first one is breech and the second cephalic (head down), it will be impossible to perform a vaginal delivery in that a condition called interlocking twins can develop, in which the head of one twin is stuck behind the chin of the other one. This can be a potentially devastating condition. If the first twin is cephalic, and the second breech or cephalic, a vaginal delivery can be attempted, provided both babies look well throughout the course of labor and have not developed any element of distress. The current trend is to have a C-section even if the circumstances are right for a vaginal birth, simply because it is safer to do so.

Despite what you may have to go through, keep in mind that you will be fortunate enough to have twice the rewards of everyone else. Or in my friends Dan and Michelle's case, four times the rewards.

I am worried about losing a lot of blood in labor. Can I give my own blood?

There is little likelihood that you will require a transfusion. The estimated risk of developing AIDS or hepatitis B/C from a common pool of blood is in the range of 1 in 250,000. It is amazing how God made us to have increased blood volume to accommodate for the potential for blood loss in delivery. If, however, you are at risk for blood loss from a clotting disorder, or if you've had a severe postpartum hemorrhage with a prior pregnancy, you can talk to your physician about arranging a family member to donate blood.

Donating your own blood may prove problematic in that it may lower your own blood volume, rendering you anemic and, therefore, un-able to supply your developing infant with the proper oxygen. If you are more comfortable with a family member donating blood, fine. But the overall risk of developing AIDS from a blood transfusion isn't any lower when the donation is from a friend or family member.

After I delivered my son, my very sexually active single brother wanted to donate blood on my son's behalf. My son was quite anemic due to having had sustained an abruption, which resulted in a lot of peripartum blood loss. Needless to say, I told him "Thanks, but no thanks." Although it was a very sweet offer, it wasn't one I was willing to risk, especially after meeting his last girlfriend.

I had a C-section in the past. Will I need a C-section again?
Your practitioner's decision to do a C-section after you have had a prior C-section is dependent upon the type of incision that was made in the uterus with the last delivery and the current circumstances of this pregnancy. Also, maternal desire to undergo a trial of labor is weighed heavily in the equation. A low transverse incision in the uterus is made whenever possible so that a vaginal delivery can be attempted with the next pregnancy. If a classical or vertical incision was made, the next pregnancy would have to result in a C-section. How successful a VBAC (vaginal birth after C-section) will be is dependent upon the reasons for the first C-section, such as whether it was done to deliver a breech baby, or due to fetal distress, or cephalopelvic disproportion (head too big for pelvis or pelvis too small for presenting part). If done for cephalopelvic disproportion, the weight of the current baby will prove helpful in assessing the potential of a vaginal birth.

Even if the second pregnancy has a baby of higher birth weight than the first, a vaginal delivery may still be feasible. This occurs 75% of the time, in that the head may accommodate the pelvis by being anterior instead of posterior, and the pubic bone may widen at the symphasis (midline where the two pelvic bones come together) more so with the second pregnancy. Because a successful vaginal birth can occur 75% of the time, physicians used to be adamant about encouraging VBAC's. Now, however, with the litigious climate being what it is, a C-section is more readily recommended. Before the patient undergoes the long, arduous task of attempting a vaginal birth, she should be made aware of the potential of needing a C-section despite her endeavors.

A repeat C-section is often met with a quicker recovery than a C-section that is performed after a long, difficult and uncomfortable labor. The benefits of having a quicker recovery after a vaginal birth, however, exceed those of a C-section. The risk of uterine rupture from the attempt at vaginal delivery is increased, as is the risk of fetal compromise. Now do you see why medicine is not black and white? It can be hell to make the best decision for you, but believe me, we try.

I have had recurrent herpes outbreaks prior to and during this pregnancy. Will I need a C-section?
There is much less likelihood of transmission of the herpes virus if one delivers vaginally in the face of recurrent outbreak than there would be if it were a primary outbreak (the first time you ever had herpes). However, because the risk of neonatal compromise is so pronounced if you did indeed have a primary outbreak and less if you have a recurrent outbreak, it is recommended that a C-section be performed in the face of an active lesion. Hopefully, if you haven't been prone to recurrences, you won't be prone to them during pregnancy.

Because pregnancy is an immune-compromised state, it is important that you eat well, rest often, drink plenty of fluids, and take your vitamins in order to avoid problems. It is now recommended that if you have a history of herpes, you should take an antiviral agent beginning around week 34 to cut down your risk of recurrence at the time of delivery.

I had spotting after sex. Does that mean I have placenta previa, and will I hemorrhage in childbirth?

The answer to that question is more than likely, no. With the advent of ultrasounds done in the second trimester, placenta location is documented early on. If your physician told you that the placenta was covering the opening of the womb at that point in time, a repeat ultrasound would have been required later in the pregnancy and the location of the placenta again assessed. The placenta migrates upward to the fundus (top portion of the uterus), where the blood supply is best; therefore, even if you had a partial previa early on in pregnancy, there is a good likelihood that it will not be present as you advance closer to term.

While there are different types of previa, a complete previa would require a C-section. A marginal previa may result in a vaginal birth pending the compression of the presenting part against the cervix and the amount of bleeding present at the time of labor. Depending on the circumstances at the time of birth, you or your practitioner might opt not to undergo a trial of labor.

Vaginal bleeding after intercourse is a common occurrence in the third trimester since the vessels in the cervix are engorged from the increased blood supply. Hence, when the penis bumps against these vessels, bleeding can occur. It is often pinkish or brownish tinged. The same scenario may occur after a vaginal exam during this time. It is not a danger sign, although it should be reported to your physician. He may advise abstinence, but be brave—that is not a reason not to report it.

Bright red bleeding or persistent spotting can be from the placenta. Even if a report of placenta previa was not made earlier in the pregnancy, it may require immediate evaluation since there could be a separation of the placenta known as an abruption.

Pink or brown-tinged, bloody mucous that is accompanied by contractions can be a sign of labor. The bloody "show" that you have often heard of can occur as a result of cervical change. As the cervix dilates, it may take mucous and blood with it, which may pass as a blood-tinged discharge or as a glob of mucous. This is no reason to run to the hospital, as labor may not occur for several days afterwards. The cervix may begin to dilate and efface prior to the onset of labor. As a matter of fact, many a woman leaves my office at 3-4 centimeters and does not go into labor for a couple of weeks afterwards. On the flip side, I may examine someone and find that her cervix is long, closed and rather thick, and she may go into labor that evening. Her labor may be longer than the woman who was 3 to 4 centimeters to begin with, but nevertheless she may get the job done sooner, if not faster.

Therefore, although the two main words in your vocabulary have become "dilated" and "effaced," labor isn't labor until the fat lady sings, and that, my dear, will be you. And believe me, you will sing in a high-pitched key you never dreamt your vocal cords were capable of reaching.

One more thought about placenta previa while we are on the subject of vaginal bleeding. If it is diagnosed early in the pregnancy, the majority of times it does abate by itself by migration. If, however, it becomes a worrisome scenario and vaginal bleeding is persistent, bed rest will become necessary, as will vaginal rest from the time the diagnosis is made until delivery. Vaginal rest means nothing in the vagina—no penis, fingers, tampons or suppositories, *nada, señorita*. And no sexual stimulation, since uterine contractions can result in vaginal bleeding from the portion of the placenta which is not adequately embedded in the uterine wall.

While vaginal rest may be a sentence for some akin to walking in a desert with no food or water, for others it will prove to be a welcome respite from the drudgery of the long-lasting, never-ending orgasm which some may have experienced in the second and early third trimester. Oh, you were not lucky enough to have one of those? Sorry, maybe next time. But remember, nothing can give you a headache like hanging out at that plateau forever.

So, when will I deliver? Am I dilated?

I often get this question at the 36-week visit, when the beta-strep culture is performed. Keep in mind before you ask this question that your physician is not a prophet or a psychic. He knows what your cervix is doing at that point in time, but foreseeing the time of delivery is quite a different story. Very often, multiparous patients (who we practitioners refer to as a multip) do not actually efface and dilate until they are in active labor. Therefore, a seemingly unfavorable cervix may prove quite favorable 24 hours later.

Patients having their first baby tend to efface and dilate prior to going into labor. Therefore, if I examine this first-time-pregnant patient (who we practitioners refer to as a primip) at 36-37 weeks and find that her cervix has thinned out quite a bit and dilated, I *may* tell that patient that she may deliver before her due date. I usually don't tell the neurotics anything, because they will hold me to it. I also am reserved about telling the whiners my predictions because they will cry if they don't deliver by the date I predicted. But again, I am often surprised at the amount of dilation and effacement that may occur without labor. Certainly the only thing I can be adamant about is whether or not the cervix is favorable enough to perform an induction of labor if the need arises.

Am I at risk for having a preterm birth?

That may be unpredictable if this is your first pregnancy. There are certain people, however, who are at risk, such as those who smoke and drink alcohol, those who gain an inadequate amount of weight, and those who have physical, emotional or psychological handicaps. Those who have taken drugs in pregnancy, have had surgery or infections during their pregnancy, or work long hours and lead stressful lives are at risk for preterm labor. Many physicians that I treat do go into preterm labor, and I warn them of this possibility early in their pregnancies. People who have a known malformation of the uterus or a fibroid uterus may also have a tendency toward preterm labor.

Preterm uterine contractions are different than preterm labor in that many uteruses are irritable and like to contract. With hydration and rest, these contractions may subside, and the cervix will not change, dilate or efface in any significant way. However, if cervical change is documented, then the diagnosis of preterm labor is made. If you are contracting before the 36th week, your practitioner will send you to labor and delivery, where you will be hooked up to a fetal monitor to assess your contractions.

These contractions can be stopped in various ways. Hydration and tocolytics (medicine that stops labor), such as Terbuteline, can result in uterine relaxation; however, this medication also works on the cardiac muscle and may cause palpitations, shortness of breath and facial flushing. These symptoms are not tolerated by some patients, so other medications may be used, such as magnesium sulfate, which also works to decrease the contractility of the uterus. This drug is reserved for those who don't tolerate Terbuteline well, in that it is given intravenously and is oftentimes done in the face of continued contractions, or if advanced dilatation is already noted when the patient does present in labor at a gestational age of less than 34-35 weeks.

Another drug is Nifedipine, also known as Procardia, which is actually used for cardiac patients and those with high blood pressure. It is a calcium antagonist and works to block the contractility of the uterus caused by the increased calcium exchange. It, too, can cause an element of hypotension, facial flushing and dizziness, but this is usually only with the first dose.

There are a number of reasons why a person goes into preterm labor. Those at risk, as mentioned earlier, are at risk because their activity or work environment or physical condition may result in an abruption or separation of the placenta from the uterus. A decreased amount of nutrition to the placental bed can result in an early maturation of the placenta and a decreased efficiency. Infections can release enzymes which also cause uterine contractions. A workup for all of the above reasons would be in order if a woman presents in preterm labor.

If a woman had preterm labor in a prior pregnancy, she may also do so with subsequent pregnancies and should be watched closely. Sometimes (as with me) a true etiology is never found—a mystery we have to live with. But other times we can use useful tests to help us predict the likelihood of occurrence. If your history in some way alerts your doctor or concerns you, we can do a fetal fibronectin (FFN) screening. This test is done with a speculum exam. A vaginal swab is used to detect a protein in the vagina only present if there has been a separation of the amniotic sac from the uterine wall. It is therefore an early indicator of labor, and it helps the practitioner to know whether or not the increase in your uterine activity will put you at risk for cervical change.

The test, like all tests, has its limitations. There are false positives, and it only gives us reassurance that you should not go into labor for at least two weeks. After that time the test would need to be repeated if you are still early enough along to warrant tocolysis. We don't want to treat you unnecessarily, but by the same token we do not want your cervix to change and put you at risk for delivering a baby whose lungs are not mature. Therefore, false positives are better than false negatives.

Another useful screen is the measurement of the cervical length, which is done via ultrasound. If the cervix looks unusually shortened or opened, your practitioner may determine it is time for bed rest and treatment. Sometimes in the case of incompetence (no, we do not think you are incompetent, we are talking about your cervix), a stitching of the cervix is recommended.

We talked about incompetence earlier when we spoke about your history. In many cases incompetence (a premature shortening or effacing and dilating of the cervix) can be detected on routine 2nd trimester ultrasound screening. It is NOT considered labor, but rather deemed as a malfunction in the muscular architecture of the cervix. The cervix is too weak to do its job of supporting the gravid uterus. In other words, it just can't shut its mouth. So the stitch, which is called a cerclage, may be recommended.

My pregnancies were complicated with preterm labor. During my first pregnancy, when I was only 27 weeks and a fourth-year resident, I was doing a vaginal hysterectomy and having continued pain on the right side of my back in the location of my kidney. I was convinced that I had a kidney stone, but I continue to work meticulously as the sweat poured down my forehead. I was a lot braver when I was young and more foolish than I am now.

When I was done with the surgery, I gave a sample of my urine, which didn't show any blood or evidence of infection. I was kind of confused as to why I was having pain. Being a fourth-year resident, I should have been astute enough to realize that these were contractions. But I was fooled because I'd never had contractions, and they were only on one side of my back.

The bottom line is, if you experience a continued pain that is colicky in nature (coming and going), gets worse as time progresses, and is occurring in a rhythmic fashion, whether it be in the front of your abdomen, in your back or one side of your abdomen, keep in mind that this could be labor, and at less than 36 weeks, it is preterm labor unless proven otherwise. If so, it usually needs to be stopped. There are some times we let a person continue laboring; for example, if the fluid is diminished or if the patient has a medical condition that requires an early delivery anyway.

Although you may be reluctant to ask your doctor about your hemorrhoids that became more aggressive over the weekend, never, ever feel awkward about calling your physician if you're experiencing these symptoms. A preterm birth can be prevented if diagnosed early.

I can't take one more day of this. What can I do?

Well, if you really want to try to deliver and you are beyond 39 weeks, I'll often recommend having sex. The prostaglandins released from the sperm can ripen the cervix (those little suckers are good for something!). If you choose to exercise this endeavor, I will refer you to one of the many books on sex and satisfying positions, and I would encourage your partner to do as many push-ups as possible, since he will need upper body strength if he chooses to be on top, and if he doesn't, God bless him. It is only the bravest of men who choose otherwise.

I'm sure you have all heard wives' tales regarding home remedies to end the never-ending pregnancy. Many patients have been told by a grandmother to eat hot and spicy Mexican or Chinese food, or to use a lot of balsamic vinegar in a dressing. Or to drink castor oil, or cod liver oil. Yuck! If you do that, the only thing you might experience is excessive burning in your anus while pushing and excessive belching while trying to breathe correctly. As you may be aware, Mexican food is made with a lot of beans; therefore, you'll never catch an obstetrician recommending it as a source of culinary pleasure at term for obvious reasons. Then again, if you're not particularly fond of your obstetrician, you may choose to eat it each evening around the time of your due date—who knows, you might get lucky and be able to blow the arrogant SOB away!

Family members may tell you to walk vigorously and go up the stairs often; however, you may actually find yourself running after all of the hot and spicy meals they have recommended! With a little pleading, once you are past your due date, you may be able to coax your physician into stripping your membranes or performing a vigorous internal exam, which may stimulate labor. If it works, labor will usually kick in within 48 hours after the exam.

While some of you may have heard about stimulating your nipples to cause labor, I caution you not to do this in that it can over-stimulate your uterus to contract, and without being on a fetal monitor, any fetal distress or decelerations in the baby's heartbeat would go unnoticed. So, while ending the pregnancy is an appealing thought, even I never succumbed to nipple rolling—but to be quite honest, I never discouraged my husband from doing it for me as I should have. If you choose to allow this activity, proceed with caution. You are allowed to turn one knob, but never two at a time. If you do, overstimulation will surely result in increased contractions.

Well, I don't know about you, but after this chapter I'm kind of ready for labor. But before that, just to ease some of your concerns, we'll head for Chapter 7, "No Way Out," to be followed by Chapter 8, "A Hard Day's Night."

Chapter 7

No Way Out

So, you think you're in labor, eh? What is this, the third time this week that you called the doctor and got sent home by a resident who looked at you with a raised eyebrow and folded arms? Despite this, you pleaded your case, stating, "I know I was feeling contractions at home!" How many times now have you awakened your partner to tell him, "Okay, this is it. It's time to go to the hospital"? By time number four, you're going to have to blast the house alarm, TV and stereo to get him out of bed, at which time he'll insist, "It's just another false alarm. Let's wait till morning." It's only after your moaning, groaning and panting that perhaps he might get the clue that this could actually be it. And if he still doesn't get the picture, you might find the need to pull a nose hair or two. If he is a pessimist, it might take a gush of fluid to soak his PJ's to convince him.

Despite the recurrent episodes of smiling nurses seeing your not-so-smiling face up on Labor & Delivery, don't be embarrassed; you're not alone. You really don't know what labor feels like, nor does anybody expect you to. Many a nurse and doctor have experienced just what you are going through. Remember me in preterm labor thinking I had a kidney stone! Just a word of caution, however. If you've had more than three visits to Labor & Delivery, you may be known as a frequent flyer. And once you are in true labor, you will be referred to as "finally having landed." Don't worry, we're all with you in your mission: to get that baby out!

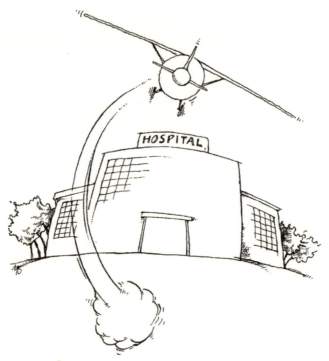

That's it! No more trips to the hospital until I see some blood, sweat and tears!

Let me preface this chapter by letting you know that we'll only talk about the first stage of labor here, which is the latent phase. This is the time that is most prolonged and least intense. At first the contractions are short and of minimal strength, so they tend not to result in too much cervical change. You may experience some episodes of indigestion and perhaps even some diarrhea. Your cramping will feel like menstrual cramps at first, then like gentle bear hugs. When the cute, innocent bear becomes a gnarling, raging grizzly, then you know it's time to show your face again. This time, it will be for real.

You may feel anticipation and excitement that may turn into fear and apprehension if this phase of labor lasts too long. If you're sent home during this phase, you may feel very sad and discouraged. A latent phase is considered prolonged if it lasts more than twenty hours in a first pregnancy, and greater than fourteen hours in a second. The contractions may not be intense enough or long enough to result in much change during that time, but believe me, they will be intense enough and long enough for you.

If you are getting wiped out, your physician may decide to stimulate labor to become more effective, or try to stop labor with narcotics such as morphine. This is known as a therapeutic rest, because it tends to be therapeutic for you, your partner, your physician, and the nurses who are caring for you. In all fairness, it does give your uterus a chance to relax and the opportunity to enter true active labor, which we will talk about in Chapter 8 when we review options for pain management.

The decision to stimulate labor or stop labor is dependent upon many factors, such as gestational age of the fetus, the well-being of the baby and you, and last but not least, the dilation and effacement of your cervix at the time that you present in latent phase labor. Also, your anxiety and discomfort will play a big role as to what your practitioner will recommend. If he thinks the time is not quite right, he may try very hard to reassure you. If there is no way to reassure you, he may deliver you with the understanding that your labor will be longer having not started from a favorable place.

What are some of the clues that labor might be coming shortly? For one, you may find yourself doing what is called nesting. This is when, several days prior to labor, you have an exceptional amount of energy and do things that you wouldn't otherwise deem necessary. For me it was cleaning. For some it might be preparing old photo albums, cutting the grass or cleaning out closets. Since I was always in preterm labor, I was constantly doing my rendition of nesting.

I like to paint, and I did so with such vehemence that I truly became the epitome of the psychotic artist that we all know or have read about. You all think Van Gogh was nuts—ha! I had it way up on him. Many of my paintings showed a bizarre and different style that I wasn't used to. When not pregnant I often paint bright and cheerful scenes, meadows, sunshine and oceans. But when I was pregnant, I began to appreciate Rembrandt's style more and more and tried to mimic his use of light in a dark and dreary room. The only problem was, I was always forgetting to put the light in.

Around this time I was constantly sending my husband out for paint, until one day he told me that my paintings were very ugly. Of course I was an emotional wreck at the time, and I decided to cry and sent him out to the store for clay so that I could sculpt. I think he must have learned his lesson, because he assured me that my sculptures were reminiscent of Michelangelo's works in his early days.

I also joined a book club and purchased every book published that year. It's no wonder my husband couldn't bear the thought of another pregnancy after having to deal with this twice in a row, but what I'm convinced really spooked him was my enrollment in the home shopping network. Now you know why we are divorced.

The next thing you may experience is the dropping of the baby into the birth canal. This occurs sooner in a first pregnancy than in subsequent ones. You might notice that you are now able to breathe easier, but like most things in life, something good is always accompanied by a compromise of sorts. Now that you're breathing great, you're constantly wetting your pants and waddling like a duck. The baby's head is so far into your pelvis that riding a Clydesdale bareback would be a piece of cake. About now you're wondering whether high heels and short skirts will ever be a part of your wardrobe again.

Often I get phone calls from patients asking me, "I have passed my mucous plug. Does that mean I'm going into labor?" The answer is no. Some people never pass the plug, so no matter how hard you look for it in your toilet and in your underwear, you may never find it. The plug is the actual passage of mucous that has clogged the opening of the birth canal for nine months. Now that the cervix is starting to dilate, the head has descended, and the cervix has begun to thin out or efface, the plug may pass. It may do so as one big glob of mucous with or without blood, hence, the so called "show," "bloody show" or "showing." It may pass as a clear, slowly-flowing, mucousy discharge. It can signal labor in the next couple of hours or in a week. Your hopes should be allayed, as it does not necessarily mean that labor is imminent.

I should warn you that the mucous plug may be referred to by a variety of different names by the old wives who have kept you busy listening to their tales. I have heard it called a bootie, a muffy and a tomato. One time a patient called me at 3 a.m. and told me that her "friend" had passed. I told her that I was quite sorry and asked her if she needed anything to calm her nerves. It wasn't until she said, "I'm not nervous, doc, I'm just happy to get this damned thing over with" that I realized she was referring to her mucous plug.

While we're on the subject of calling doctors at 3 a.m., please be clear and concise with your explanation of your problems at that time, since many of us are in a sound sleep. You can do amazing things, such as answer the phone, dial phone numbers and even talk to patients, while in that state of slumber. There are certain words that doctors are tuned into which wake them out of that state, such as blood, fluid, pain and contractions. Words like muffy and bootie just don't do it.

Leaking of the membranes may occur prior to actual labor. When it does occur, you should notify your physician and go to the hospital so that you and the baby do not develop an infection. If you are past 36 weeks when the rupture occurs, you will have more than likely gotten your beta strep results. If they were positive, we would want you to go to the hospital right away to begin your antibiotics. If they were negative, we still want to know that you have ruptured so we can keep tabs on you and how long it takes you to wander over to the hospital.

If it is your first pregnancy and you are a neurotic or a wimp, you will be there in no time. If you are laid back and experienced, we would want you there no later than 5-6 hours after you ruptured, because the chance of other infections, despite a negative strep culture, still exist. If you are less than 36 weeks, we want you there so that we can start antibiotics, since we don't know your beta strep results and need to treat you as though you are positive to avoid infection.

Rupturing of the membranes can occur in the obvious fashion with a large gush of fluid. This will no doubt happen in public, like while you are shopping in the grocery store, causing you to slip and slide down the aisle. Or you may experience a trickle that you can't stop no matter how hard you try to cross your legs and tighten your buns. Either way, it is important that you note the color of the fluid and time of rupture so that your physician will know whether it is necessary to augment (stimulate) your labor if you don't do it on your own.

Prior to the actual labor, the biggest question on most patients' minds is, "How do I differentiate fake from active labor?" In other words, "How do I avoid making a total fool of myself?" Don't worry, it's impossible not to make a fool of yourself. If you ruptured your water it is easy; you don't have to speculate about labor, that is, unless you just wet your pants with pee pee and didn't know it. Then we are talking major fool. Not really, just kidding. It happens all the time. And if you are unsure if you've peed your pants, we want to know you are unsure. We would rather check to be sure than run the risk of infection. Sometimes it is just plain hard to tell.

Fake labor oftentimes is down low, above the pubic bone or above the hairline, which feels like a constant cramping that is very difficult to time. It may come and go and last for 20-30 seconds. It is never pleasant feeling, but it in no way is intense enough to result in excessive pain or discomfort, or cervical change, for that matter.

NINE MONTHS TO GO

True early or latent phase of labor starts at the top of the uterus, which is just under your breastbone. Often you'll feel a knot-like sensation that wraps around your back and then goes down into your groin. It feels almost as though you were being hugged by a sumo wrestler. It doesn't hurt, and it may feel somewhat soothing and comforting at first (like maybe the first two contractions, and then the comfort stuff goes right out the window).

How you know you're getting more active and closer to the real thing is that this soothing sensation turns into a sharper, persistent pain, making you aware that the sumo wrestler is suddenly angry that he doesn't have any balls. The pains may become sharper and be closer and closer together. They will be of longer and longer duration—upwards of 40 to 60 seconds, occurring every 2-3 minutes instead of every 5-8 minutes. It may become more intense, to the point where you may feel that pain medication is a much better option than walking around at home.

Under no circumstances are you to drive yourself to the hospital! The ride to the hospital will be threatening enough—especially to your significant other, who is suddenly thinking about not being so significant. I can attest to the fact that a marriage must be mighty strong if a couple comes in holding hands in active labor.

Another question I am asked is, "What should I bring to the hospital?" Pack light. Pack light. Pack light! Especially since you're probably going to have your partner carry that bag in and out of the hospital at least three times. Also, while you're laboring you are not going to want to wear your newest nightie from Victoria's Secret. Labor and delivery tend to be quite a messy experience for everyone involved. Which reminds me, if you like your socks, don't wear them. If your partner likes his shoes, tell him to wear another pair.

Even if you are a perfect priss, you need very little while in the hospital. If you pack a heavy bag, you will find it sitting on your lap in the wheelchair by the fourth trip to the hospital. And believe me, you already have way too much on your lap to have that heavy thing to deal with. Be kind to your partner and he will be kind to you.

Once you get to the hospital, you will receive a lovely hospital gown which will be loosely placed so that a fetal monitor can assess your contraction activity and the baby's heartbeat. Two tocos (receptors that will pick up contraction intensity and fetal heart rate)—that's tocos, not tacos—will be attached to straps that will be attached to your abdomen and to a monitor. Imagine the wonderful feeling of having these straps on you as you're feeling the cramping of yet another contraction.

Once you are all plugged in and ready to fly, it is at this point in time that they will send your partner or labor coach down to admissions. Assuming that you have pre-registered, he has very little to do, and since he has a lot on his mind right now, we hope to keep it that way.

After you have been on the monitor for a while, an OB resident (if you are in a teaching hospital) or OB nurse may come in to check you to see if your cervix is making any favorable changes and, therefore, to determine whether or not you need be sent home (yet again) or have the luxury of staying in this facility, which you now have become very accustomed to, assuming, of course, you fall under the common category of "frequent flyer." This term is used with the greatest love and respect. Believe me, we feel for you.

If you do get to stay, you'll find out just how dilated and effaced you are. Don't get too excited. Remember, first labors can be quite long. Also remember that you may be contracting, but your cervix may not be at all that ripe and, therefore, you may be sent home to walk or to relax and come back when you're more active and the contractions are closer together. I send many of my patients to the mall, which is in close proximity to our office, as is Walmart—aren't we lucky? I feel that while they are in pain, they at least deserve to do something nice, like shop. I felt that I deserved to shop when I was in preterm labor. I even rented a wheelchair and managed to find different people to push me around the mall. And my husband thought he was safe with me on bed rest—HA! I showed him.

If you are sent home, don't be discouraged as you may be in early labor, and it is always better to manage that part of labor at home in your own environment or at the mall spending money. As long as you haven't ruptured the bag of water, and the baby is moving and you're not too uncomfortable, being home might actually make the labor more tolerable. Time in the hospital can prove to be annoying.

Many residents, interns and medical students feel an overwhelming desire to introduce themselves to you in case they are present for your delivery. You might have an early IV, which is fluid given intravenously. You might be the subject of lengthy questioning by the interns and residents, which can be a little difficult if you know you have many more hours to spend there seeing everyone's smiling face. And after your little "outdoor" adventure, you may return and be 2-3 centimeters dilated, 75% thinned out, and the head may be well against the cervix, which qualifies you as a keeper. Finally, you have now landed.

Once the resident that you spit at hours ago tells you this, your natural instincts make you want to jump out of bed and do the moon dance; but you compose yourself, realizing how funny it would look to everyone, and how easily you could slip and fall, yet again making an ass of yourself.

Okay, guys. You're in latent phase labor. You're on your way to active phase. You're happy as a lark. You know you're staying, and you're sucking on a lollipop and smiling at your partner. You have gotten a dose of narcotics through the vein to take the edge off the discomfort that is now starting to mount. You think labor is a piece of cake and that the contractions are not that hard, and you might even do this naturally. HA! And all your friends told you otherwise. Next chapter, Active Labor. You'll be asking for those pain meds, and they'll be waiting for you!

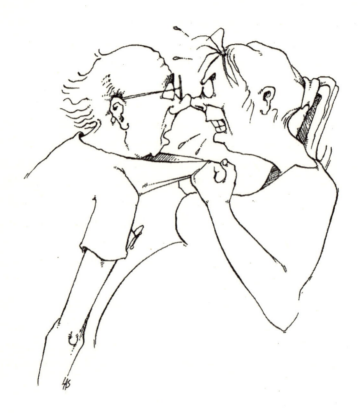

Listen Doc, give me my epidural now or you'll wish you were a proctologist!

Chapter 8

A Hard Day's Night

You're in active labor, and for some reason, although it's 3 o'clock in the morning, you're extremely hyper and alert. You're hooked up to the monitor and the nurse starts an IV. You can deal with this pain because right now you're as happy as can be that you're actually here and staying! For some reason the lyrics of a Beatles song keep popping into your head, and you agree it's a hard day's night. You also think, as you hum away, that you can handle anything—you are woman, hear you roar, and we will—you're invincible, and you're one third of the way there.

You tell your nurse with glee, "I'll be doing this without the epidural, thank you very much." She looks at you and smirks. You think to yourself that she must be a wimp. But I'll remind you, ladies, don't be rash—not even you, Miss Priss—because remember, it ain't over till the fat lady sings, and you do remember who that is, don't you?

Once your doctor has examined you and determined that you are in labor, he may break your bag of water, which will inevitably speed labor up. Following this you will soon be in transition (phase 3 of labor). What this means is that you have gone from the latent (early) phase of labor to the active phase of labor. What that means to you and your loved ones is that you are no longer the sweet kitten that you were in early labor—smiling and thankful that you were there, appreciative that you got your ice chips, and all apologetic that you were laughing and silly after you were given your IV narcotics.

You have undergone a major transition. You are now a witch who has lost her broom, a man-eating tiger who hasn't smelled prey in over a month, or a dog without a bone. Your partner has now seen you in a different light, one that is much darker than ever before. You're using language he has only heard in boot camp or at a construction site of an inner-city skyscraper. We doctors and nurses know how to detect the subtle signs of true labor. It is at this time we may be called to check to see if your progress warrants an epidural. Believe me, you're not the only one who's praying that it's time to get one!

Let's just spend a couple of minutes now and review the history of pain relief in labor. In the early 1800s Dr. Simpson gave a laboring woman chloroform after she had a difficult time while pushing. When she woke up she didn't believe she had given birth. She was depressed about not having experienced this climactic event (in my opinion, she was truly psychotic). Dr. Simpson had accomplished what the field of medicine had hoped to achieve in labor: the elimination of pain without doing harm to the mother or fetus.

At first there was great debate over the relief of pain. It was considered immoral by the clergy, since a woman was "meant" to bear pain due to Eve's indiscretion. Who says this is not a chauvinistic world in which we live? Did they have selective amnesia? I mean, she just handed him the damn apple—he was the one stupid enough to bite!

In the 1950s and 1960s women started becoming more independent. They began to feel that the experience of labor would be better enjoyed rather than endured. (Hence was born the end of martyrdom.) Finally, the field of medicine, because of its strong and never-ending desire to meet the needs and comfort of its patients, developed a mechanism with which relief of labor could be accomplished while the experience was acute and tangible. Hence, the spinal and epidural came to be.

Indications for pain relief are:

1) a long labor in which the mom is unable to tolerate the pain.

2) the inability of a patient to push effectively because of her increased discomfort.

3) the need for the use of forceps or a complicated delivery.

4) if the obstetrician is repeatedly kicked, wounding him and making it difficult for a successful delivery.

5) the need for C-section due to the inability to progress in labor or due to fetal distress.

6) my favorite reason. You want it and you're ready, both emotionally and physically.

You are now in transition and your cervix is starting to change. If a patient is in active labor and very uncomfortable, other forms of pain relief may be attempted prior to an epidural. The reason for attempting other forms of pain relief could be that the cervix is not dilated enough, or perhaps the patient does not want an epidural. It is our job to both enlighten her and respect her wishes.

Tranquilizers can be offered in the early part of labor. These drugs, such as Phenergan and Vistaril, are used to relax and calm the anxious patient. There are times they work very well throughout the whole labor, making an epidural unnecessary (it is rare). They are most often used in the early active phase of labor. They enhance the effectiveness of analgesics such as Demerol and Stadol. There are some women who like the effects these medications have on them, and others who feel a loss of control or loss of memory. The number of times they are used throughout labor depends on the progress a patient is making in labor and how well she tolerated or got relief from the medication.

Acupuncture, acupressure and reflexology. I am a firm believer in the effectiveness of western medicine, except when it comes to labor management. The last thing you want when you are uncomfortable is to be poked or prodded. Of course, I may be biased, because I tried acupuncture for my carpel tunnel at first, and all it did for me is make me have more pain. I was told I was too sensitive. And as far as reflexology, my feelings are that putting pressure on my little feet is in no way going to relieve the God awful pain from my large contracting uterus. But if you want to try it, go for it. Hopefully it won't be too late to get your epidural after you spent an hour having somebody rub your feet. Your feet might feel good anyway.

Hypnobirthing. Sorry, folks, I have been doing this stuff for 22 years and I have NEVER seen it work. I have seen lots of people try it. Some people even have hypnotherapists with them in labor. If you are into yoga, and if you have practiced various techniques for relaxation, or if your labor goes exceedingly fast, it might work. I am, however, a skeptic about this, simply because I haven't seen much success. Part of its effectiveness, though, is believing that it works, so if you want it to work, don't believe me!

Epidural. This is what 75% of women choose. It is popular because in experienced hands, it is safe. Local pain relief is given, but the patient is still able to move and be awake and not groggy throughout the remaining (more uncomfortable) part of labor. Yes, it is injected around the spinal cord. But it goes into the space between the ligaments that surround the membrane covering the spinal cord. In other words, there is no risk of paralysis, as you may have heard from ole Aunt Mary.

If you decide on the epidural, your doctor will need to be sure you are not dehydrated. If you are, then the medication can lower your blood pressure. So an IV is started and fluid is given to you prior to the anesthesiologist's being called. If labor is slowed, Pitocin can be started (this is a form of the hormone that triggers the uterus to contract), and yes, you can push with an epidural. Yepeeee!

NINE MONTHS TO GO

Before the obstetrician gives the epidural to the patient, he must make sure that labor is progressing adequately. You do not have to be dilated beyond 3-4 centimeters, you just need to be in active labor. We like to avoid the epidural in latent phase labor if at all possible because if given too early, it may slow down labor or even shut down the effective response of the uterus to contract. We can give a patient Pitocin, which would make the uterus contract effectively, but we wind up playing catch-up for many hours in some instances. Therefore, the time frame in which the epidural is given is quite important.

The epidural has minimal side effects, yet gives effective pain relief. It doesn't eliminate the perception of labor, but decreases its intensity significantly enough so that labor can be experienced. It is the optimum pain relief since, if given at the right time, it doesn't lengthen the course of labor.

Naturally, I had to experience labor so that I could adequately explain the wondrous event to my patients. I experienced two contractions in active phase, and then was quite adamant about receiving my epidural when I was only 2 centimeters dilated. When I kindly asked my husband to go out and tell the anesthesiologist that I was ready, he said to me, "Now, Joann, don't take labor into your own hands. Remember, you're the patient here, not the doctor." I seem to remember him saying that on several occasions; however, that time I grabbed his shirt, drew him close to me and strangled him. He was nice and quiet after that and a good little coach—or was that after I pulled the hairs out of his right forearm? If you like your FOB (father of the baby) and hope to stay with him to help raise your new child, get your epidural early.

As far as questions about active labor, I will take the liberty to answer what some of you may ask. However, to be perfectly honest, by the time you're asking for pain relief, you won't give a damn about anything but when and how your pain will go away. But in fairness to those of you who are less wimpy than myself, I will proceed to those questions that might be asked, and to emphasize their importance, I will word them according to the way many of my patients have done in the past.

FREQUENTLY ASKED QUESTIONS

What the hell can I have for pain?

I think I have answered this question already, but for those of you who are a little denser, I will reiterate. Demerol and Vistaril or Nuban and Phenergan are powerful combinations that can be given in an IV. They can also be given as a shot in your butt, or both. The decrease in pain and relief varies widely from patient to patient. Therefore, in early labor this is an attempted option prior to giving an epidural. A sensitive patient may become nauseous and vomit. We never like to give these drugs while a patient is pushing because there is a minimal crossing of the placenta, and the baby may be respiratorally depressed. Therefore, it is the preferable option for early labor.

Some patients become giddy and silly when given narcotics. I was one such patient. My future business partners who were delivering me had given me the Stadol and then talked to me about the stipulations in the new contract. Of course, those bums knew I would say yes to anything, and they were right.

What can I have to decrease my anxiety?

Tranquilizers may be given, such as Vistaril or Phenergan, to calm you and decrease your level of anxiety. Again, for the reasons mentioned above, these are usually given early in labor.

You can hire a doula. It wouldn't do it for me, but go for it if you want; you can always fire her. "Doula" is a term that comes from ancient Greece. It was a female servant. Her primary role is a continuous, never-ending source of comfort, support and encouragement. In other words, she does everything your lazy ass partner should be doing. She helps with those useful relaxation techniques we talked about. She will also get you your ice chips and rub your back. A good doula will not let your partner feel left out. If you want a doula, you probably will be well suited for a midwife delivery. She will be best at augmenting the support of the doula.

Most doctors find their techniques a little annoying, at least I and my partners do. I suppose I really shouldn't speak for other doctors. The reason we tend to feel this way is that many of the doulas we have encountered are so adamant about the patient "doing it naturally" that if the patient chooses otherwise she is made to feel like a failure. However, like with everything in life, there is good and bad. Research your doula and make sure she will not talk you out of something you really might want. For those of you who are doulas, I am sorry if I insulted you. I am sure you serve a very important service for all the wimpy whiners out there that we all know and love.

What are some other options for pain relief? What is a nerve block? Will it make me less nervous?

A nerve block is an anesthetic injected along the course of the nerves. It is used to deaden sensation in the intended region for which it is given. It may be used for a surgical delivery (C-section) or for the use of forceps. A regional block, also known as an epidural or spinal, is perfect because Mom can remain awake during the birth experience and afterwards, even in the event of a C-section.

Sometimes the urge to push may be diminished after an epidural, and for a short time the patient may be unable to push effectively. The dose of the medicine may need to be decreased for a more adequate second stage of labor, which is the pushing phase. Nowadays we use a constant drip infusion to administer the medication through a catheter. The luxury of the constant infusion is you never have to feel pain to know you need more medication. Ideally, when the therapeutic range is reached, it can be maintained and then diminished if a patient is pushing poorly in the second stage of labor. If the anesthetic decreases the effectiveness of contractions, it can be easily rectified by decreasing the anesthetic or by adding oxytocin (Pitocin).

The epidural is given often and is very safe and easy to administer. Other blocks include the pudendal, spinal or caudal block. I tend not to use blocks in the second stage of labor while pushing because all it accomplishes is that you get a numb butt and still have pain. I like the epidural because it allows the patient to be comfortable while pushing and also allows me to repair the vagina (episiotomy) without being yelled at or kicked. It also makes for adequate relaxation of the perineum and vaginal muscles in the event that an emergent vacuum and/or forceps delivery becomes necessary.

It is important to have IV fluids before an epidural is given so that one does not have a drop in blood pressure. Initial administration of the dose can cross the placenta and can have a transient effect of decreasing the fetal heart rate. Again, this is an easily rectified situation, and it is not a reason to opt for pain.

A spinal is good for a C-section, or in rare circumstances, for a forceps/vacuum delivery. I find it most useful in a patient who opted not to have any anesthesia, but is suddenly in need of rapid forceps delivery, since a spinal works very quickly and effectively. It totally limits the ability of a patient to push, however, and can only be given when the obstetrician deems pushing not to be a requirement, or if surgical intervention such as a C-section is the means of delivery. It may also affect blood pressure, but once again, that is an easily rectified situation.

General anesthesia is used in the case of an emergent need to perform an operative intervention, such as a C-section in the case of fetal distress. The disadvantage is that the woman doesn't experience the wonderful climax of giving birth.

If all else fails, there is always the use of hypnotism and yoga in non-operative deliveries and labor. They have both been proven effective. You must, however, be capable to concentrate on placing mind over matter. Although you may have mastered this feat in early pregnancy, it now may prove to be a grueling and exhausting endeavor because your matter is so much more than it once was. Therefore, if you choose this option despite my beliefs, you should work with a certified hypnotist in early pregnancy so that you will be better able to increase the capability of that mind of yours.

The TENS unit (transcutaneous electrical nerve stimulation) is a means of giving stimulation to the sensory nerve inputs along the nerve pathways of the areas in question. I have yet to see it work in labor. Acupuncture works along the same principles as does the TENS unit; however, you're using needles instead of stimulation, and most doctors are not trained in this procedure.

Personally, I as a physician might find it very hard to concentrate on my task as I watch the patient push with needles sticking out of odd places and various body parts. It may also prove to be a liability. When the patient pushes, she needs to tighten various muscles. If you use your imagination, you can see how the tightening and relaxation involved in pushing could dislodge one of the needles. It certainly wouldn't be a pretty sight if as you pushed, one of those guys sprung loose, flew out and hit your obstetrician in the head, therefore making your delivery even more difficult than you had anticipated.

The last option is distraction and/or massage given by a therapist, friend or spouse. If you choose this option, keep in mind that the friend or spouse you have chosen may no longer exist as such after you deliver.

You should discuss options of labor management with your practitioner long before you enter labor. Find out what his belief system is and how willing he is to rid you of your pain in labor. Is he liberal or conservative in his approach? If you wish to be brave and go through this ordeal without assistance, communicate this to him. Never close your mind to alternatives. You really don't know what it feels like, nor do any of us expect you to. Realize that just because your Grandma Brunhilda delivered on a mountain top in a clover patch, as the billy goat next to her watched eagerly, you should not let these pre-conceived, idealistic notions about labor make your decision. What should be most important to you is the safety and well-being of you and your baby.

Can I walk with my epidural?

Sure, if you want to fall down. Actually, there are some institutions that offer the so-called walking epidural. We don't. We feel that once the patient is uncomfortable enough to be given an epidural, she is too wiped out to get up and aimlessly wander the halls. Besides, we feel that monitoring the baby is safer during that active phase of labor. If you truly find the need to get up, ask your practitioner if the anesthesiologist at your hospital offers this form of pain relief. The walking epidural is similar to the fast-acting spinal block that is used in a single dose for an emergent delivery or a C-section. It is injected into the spinal fluid, but a catheter is also then inserted into the epidural space, where a smaller amount of medicine is delivered than in the case of a regular epidural. In actuality it is a combination of the two techniques.

When will this be over? How much longer am I going to have to take this crap?

Well, keep in mind that the average first labor is anywhere between 14 and 16 hours. A multiparous patient can assume that if her labor was 14 hours the first time, it will be 7 to 10 the second time—but that's a rough rule of thumb. If your mom and/or sisters had relatively easy and quick labors, you too may have a quick one. But there are unforeseen circumstances that may result. Remember, too, that with an epidural you may push a little bit longer, but at least you'll be comfortable. The average first-time mom pushes from 1 to 2 hours.

Will I need a C-section after going through this whole damn labor?

There are many variables that may exist in any particular delivery. For example, the baby may develop an element of fetal distress. You may have CPD (cephalopelvic disproportion), meaning that although you progressed adequately in labor, the baby fails to descend into your pelvis because of the shape of the baby's head, or the position in which he came into the birth canal. Your pelvis may be too small to accommodate this shaped head. Although we readily do ultrasounds for the estimation of fetal weight, it is not always predictive of a successful vaginal birth, although it could certainly help us determine the likelihood of needing a C-section.

More than likely, before you went into labor your practitioner discussed with you the estimated size of your baby and the potential for having a shoulder dystocia. If your estimate was high, based on your weight gain, your height, the baby's estimated weight, and your risk of gestational diabetes, then you would have been offered a C-section and would not be asking this question.

If your risk was moderate and you opted for a trial at vaginal birth, both you and your practitioner know that turning in the towel in the face of minimal cervical change over a prolonged time would be more readily recommended than putting you through continued agony over time. If your heart, for some odd reason, is set on an attempt at vaginal birth—i.e. you are a sadomasochist who enjoys intense pain—then your practitioner may allow you to continue labor, with the understanding that it may not result in a successful vaginal outcome.

Unfortunately, the need for a C-section cannot always be foreseen in early labor. Sometimes the baby's position dictates success or failure. Sometimes estimated weights are not accurate. The estimation of weight can be plus or minus a pound, and when you are talking babies there is a big difference between 7 pounds 5 ounces and 8 pounds 5 ounces.

If your baby was breech prior to the attempt at labor, then at some point a version may have been attempted. If it failed, you may have been scheduled for a C-section. If, however, you presented in labor prior to the scheduled date of that version, then a C-section would need to be performed. Don't consider a C-section a defeat, especially if you labored and need to go the extra step. Remember, when this decision is made, it is made because it is what's best for you and the baby. In the future, when you're old and gray, and your friends do pee-pee in their panties while they're waiting in line at the casino to get on the big bus home, you might actually be thankful that your vagina and bladder were spared the ordeal of pushing in labor!

Well now, you're approaching that second stage of labor. That means the physician has checked you and you're now ready to push. I know you thought you were ready to push when you came in at 1 centimeter feeling all that hellish pressure, but no such luck. We are now hour 12 from when this whole thing started, and trust me, 14 hours is not bad!

You've had an undue amount of pressure despite the epidural, and your physician has checked you and found you to be complete, meaning 10 centimeters dilated. You may feel like you need to have a bowel movement, but your doctor tells you, "No, that's the baby's head." You may insist you need a bedpan, but your doctor tells you that you are ready to start pushing. Suddenly you need a refresher course. You know that you got that certificate upon completion of the birthing class, but you can't remember a damn thing. "What was that they said about breathing?"

You have a good coach. One who stands near you and is supportive, one who rubs your back, breathes with you, relaxes with you in between contractions, and if he's real good, he'll need to deal with his own hemorrhoids the next day for pushing so effectively with you. But if you don't have a good coach, fear not—the nurses and the physician are well versed and will help you with this second stage of labor. That is what we do best. So please don't be anxious. You are finally here and will meet your baby real soon.

You know that the physician is talking to you at this point, but you seem to find it very hard to remain calm and attentive to his instructions. Your coach tends to repeat the instructions to you, but you're less tolerant of him and you tell him to shut the hell up! All you remember is that your nurse told you to listen to the instructions and it will be a piece of cake. You think, "What kind of cake? Black forest, devil's food, minced meat maybe?"

NINE MONTHS TO GO

You may be wondering if you'll need an episiotomy at this time. An episiotomy, for those of you who don't know, is a surgical incision in the muscular area of your perineum between your vagina and your anus. Its purpose is to enlarge the vaginal opening. The need for an episiotomy is often times unforeseen. It's hard to say if you will or will not need one until you're actually pushing and the physician is able to see how well the perineum thins out in response to the head's coming against it.

An episiotomy is not routine. Everyone's anatomy is different, and sometimes the baby's head is too big to pass through the vagina without an episiotomy. If we think that you may tear into the rectum or the urethra (the opening of the bladder), then an episiotomy will be performed. Massaging prior to or during labor may help somewhat, but it truly depends on your anatomy, genetics and built-in elasticity that will adequately "give," so to speak, to the size and shape of the presenting part.

Since we're on the subject of episiotomies, I might say that I can't tell you how often a partner asks me to put an extra stitch in for him while I'm sewing up his wife, who just went through this long and difficult ordeal. The funny part is, they always think they are the first ones who ever said it. My inclination is to say if it's a snug fit you're looking for, things could work as easily and even better if you allow me to put a stitch at the base of your package!

Okay, guys, it's time to push. The wimpy whiners tend to be the worst pushers. They're too busy moaning and groaning to really bear down and get things over with. The laid-back experienced types will not want you to count or coach her because she prefers to do her own thing. She will push in a dimly lit room with Yanni playing piano in the stereo behind her hospital bed. She will be in control. The career-oriented neurotics, on the other hand, will really start getting nervous and hyper because they feel as though they are losing control. This is something they have never done before, and they don't want to make a mistake. After all, they usually never make mistakes.

The perfect priss is the absolute worst when it comes to pushing, because she is afraid of making poopies in front of her doc and her partner. She is worried about not doing a good job and has an overwhelming phobia of her partner looking at her vagina to see the baby's hairy head. She is fearful of what that perspective will do to her partner's perception of her once beautiful vajayjay, so she has a compulsion to constantly close her legs while pushing, which you can well imagine could make our job quite difficult. The perfect priss may also prove to be less modest than she would have been in her non-pregnant state. She might want a C-section to get this over with, since pushing makes her sweaty. However, if she concentrates and works hard, even she can push.

The doctor must take all these various forms of apprehension into account. He must find words of comfort and encouragement. The physician's and caretaker's job is to help you minimize the amount of pain you are in so that you can work together to end the situation in a favorable and productive manner. Keep in mind that the end product will be forever worth it.

No matter what type character you are, remember that pushing generally takes awhile. The more effective you are at it, the faster this whole thing comes to an end. And believe me, it will. The epidural and narcotics gave you a chance to rest up and get your strength back. Now we need you to help fight the fight. And *you can do it!* So it is now time to get over it and get to work, and if you have a hard time with that concept, just take a minute to think about the word "labor." If it was going to be a walk in the park, perhaps it would be called "picnic."

I'm convinced that the Chinese have the ancient art of labor down to a science. Many a Chinese patient that I have delivered squatted while pushing. It gave them the power to push the head out while they managed to balance themselves in that awkward position without toppling over and hitting their head. Of course, my inclination was to follow them around with a bucket, but I refrained from that and soon realized that if I didn't bother them, they would be content and do a very efficient job.

As far as people in the delivery room, I find that it is often the career-oriented neurotic that wishes to have a room full of many faces, which I'm often times surprised at, but it is their family's chance to see them differently. Warning: if you let too many people in the room, you might hear about your behavior for years and years to come. Most often birthing centers have a restriction on the number of guests, so you might luck out even if everyone is bugging you to see you make a fool of yourself. Trust me, no matter what your persuasion, ethnicity, beliefs or patient character-type, you can and will make a fool of yourself. This is a time when modesty no longer exists. It flew out the window when your mucous plug went down the drain.

If you are dead against pushing and want an elective C-section, remember that a C-section isn't without risks. Even though you may bypass the need for labor and pushing, and ultimately save the vagina (Long live the vagina! You wait—someday that will be the motto in the retirement homes throughout the nation), the baby doesn't have the luxury of his little lungs being squeezed like they are as he descends in the birth canal. The lack of this squeezing can cause a buildup of amniotic fluid and mucous in the nasal passageways and lungs, which can result in the baby aspirating (breathing in) fluid and having short-lived but frightening respiratory problems. Although this respiratory condition is usually very easily taken care of, it causes unnecessary anxiety and worry for the new parents when their newborn has to be observed in the special care nursery.

The mother can get an infection with a C-section and can actually bleed more than after a vaginal birth. Major surgery also cuts major muscles and causes a delayed recuperation. Therefore, if this approach can be avoided, it is advisable to do so. The bottom line is, nothing in life is without its risks. If you help and push as effectively as you can, not only will the job get done sooner, but it will get done with less risks and potential complications. So don't worry about your frazzled hair or poor makeup job or smelly armpits. Just go for it and bear down.

How do I push?

Here or in China? You will need to be in a semi-sitting position. You will pull your thighs back toward your chest, and your partner will hold your neck to support your chin being bent forward to make your body resemble a C shape. In other words, you will look like a squashed toad. You will bear down as you would during a bowel movement (now you know why your modesty flew out the window). Don't worry if you actually do have a bowel movement; if you do, you're using all the right muscles. And it might be a good way to get your mother-in-law out of the room. Those who truly love you will stick it out, and the rest are not worth a dump. So go ahead and have one. If nothing else, it may determine your destiny.

The instructor may tell you that you're going to take three pushes with each contraction, bearing down each time for a 10-second count. I often tell my patients to come right back in between each push, and to make the second of the three pushes the most effective. Most of us tend to push our abdominal muscles or shoulder muscles more so than our vaginal muscles. It is an exercise you can practice prior to actually pushing if you like; however, your instructor will work with you in helping you identify these muscles. If you want to practice you can do Kegel exercises, or you can put your two fingers in your vagina and practice pushing them out. Try to avoid your clitoris unless you have some time to kill. It is important that you hold your breath while pushing, and don't let any air out as you bear down. I tell my patients to keep their mouth closed —no spitting allowed. Now you know why physicians wear goggles and masks.

If you choose not to have an epidural or if your labor is moving along quite quickly, you may feel an overwhelming burning sensation as you bear down. However, if you push through that pain it will actually ease your discomfort and make for more effective pushing. Sometimes your physician may want to check you while pushing. He might ask if it is okay to check you with the next contraction. You might want to respond, "Sure, if it's okay if I squeeze your testicles with my next contraction as you do so." But actually, he is doing this for a reason. He is not trying to be malicious or cause you undue pain; he is enabling you to focus and concentrate on the location and duration of your push.

At some point your physician will tell you that the head is crowning, and you may be able to ease up on your pushing and bear down slowly. Some patients like to observe this by looking in a mirror. Others are horrified to do so and prefer closing their eyes as they bear down. Once the physician says, "No more pushing," and the baby finally comes out, you will have an overwhelming sense that this was all worth it.

To this day, I am always grateful for the opportunity to be able to deliver a child and place it on its mom's abdomen, and I am forever thankful that God, in this way, has enabled me to be close to Him by realizing each and every day the magnitude of His creations (so you see I am a caring and sensitive person, despite what you may have thought as a result of reading this book).

Although most of the time the actual delivery is quite a beautiful experience, it can seem barbaric at times. For example, there are times when a vacuum cup may need to be applied and the child may come out looking like a conehead. There are times when the baby's little face may look bruised because of the rapid descent or because of having a nuchal cord (umbilical cord around its neck), and there are times when the baby's face and lips may be swollen from having presented into the pelvis in a occiput posterior, or looking-up, position. The baby may appear bloody and may have an abundance of fine hair distributed over his or her entire body. No, that night you conceived the moon was not full and your lover did not turn into a werewolf. This is known as lanugo and is quite common.

Despite all this, you as the mother will see only beauty, and rightly so. Don't feel that you're abnormal, however, if you look at this beautiful creature as a stranger and think, "Oh, he is kind of ugly." It may take a while for you to grow accustomed to the fact that you're now a mother. Remember that birth, although a beautiful experience, is harder than running a marathon and can prove to be somewhat exhausting for both you and your baby. Give yourself a chance to adjust to the whole thing.

Once the placenta is removed, your will breathe a sigh of relief. Your uterus will then be massaged, your episiotomy and/or vaginal tears will be repaired, and the baby will be cleaned off and given back to you to love and to hold. In other words, he will no longer look like a mangy, bloody mongrel. The baby's weight is either given to you then or after the baby has gone to the nursery.

It is now time for the bonding. Of course, some avid enthusiasts put the bloody, hairy baby right onto your nipple for nursing, but think about it—after an intense workout, do you really feel like eating? Give the kid a break and let him breathe a little first. Also, after all the blood, sweat and tears you just went through, do you want something sucking yet more fluid out of your poor, stressed-out body?

Of course, this is my own bias, but in my opinion you are not odd if you don't feel like having a little one hanging off of your nipple the second after you give birth. Have some down time—gel out. Get your legs out of the stirrups first. Bonding can be done without feeding. Life can be maintained for a relatively long time without food. This is true even if you are of Italian persuasion. The last thing you may need is nipple pain in addition to the neck pain you have from pushing, the crotch pain you now have from your episiotomy, and the new onset of thigh aching from being in stirrups. Do you really want the baby hanging off your breast as you're sitting on your bag of ice to help your labial swelling? I don't think so.

It is understandable if you're not quite ready. Remember, the age of martyrdom is over, and you're not alone. Soon enough you'll be ready to nurse, change diapers and receive visitors. You may actually find yourself resenting the fact that everyone is paying such

NINE MONTHS TO GO

attention to the baby and not to you, especially since you've been through such an ordeal. With this in mind, let's head over to our final chapter, "Blue Moon."

Joann Richichi

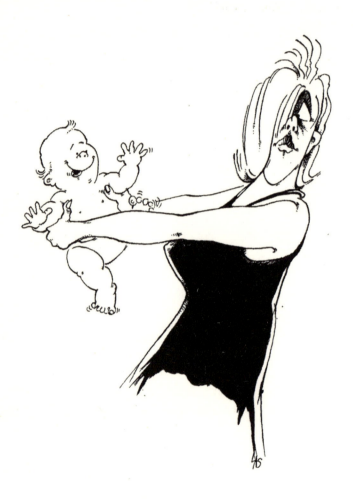

Oh, God, is it time for the next feeding already?

Chapter 9

Blue Moon

Obviously, judging by the title of this chapter, it is not meant to appeal to those of you who, after you have given birth, rush home, invite the world to see your baby, cook a seven-course meal, bake cookies and watch every episode of *Sesame Street* and *Barney* as you sing to your newborn baby. It is not meant for those of you who are in awe at all the baby can do when in fact all he can do is cry, eat and poop. Realistically speaking, at present your baby's most interesting characteristic and best assets in life are based on the shape, size and consistency of his stools, which are now quite a bit smaller than they will be soon, and much less foul than they will be once he's off his formula.

Rather, this chapter is meant for those of you who think you're weird for not having the excited enthusiasm that enables you to feel like floating on air, wanting to fly a kite or go bungee jumping. It's for those of you who are now home, and although you have a beautiful baby to look at, love and hold, you can't seem to see the light the future will hold. I don't care who you are or what patient category you may fit in. You are not alone in facing the rift that postpartum depression can cause in your life. You seem not to be focusing on your baby's beautiful face, but rather on your megarrhoids and stretch marks that all the Vitamin E in the world will not diminish.

You still feel unattractive, and you hate your partner. You can only avoid having sex for so long—you ask your doctor to tell your husband 4 months. You feel dry and jumpy and are not in the mood to be touched. Not to mention the fact that nothing fits. You feel fat and ugly and overwhelmed.

You tell yourself over and over again that you should be proud of yourself and of all your accomplishments. But then old Aunt Ethel comes over, who used to hug and hold you whenever she visited, and now she walks right past you, grabs your baby and kisses him and doesn't even ask how you feel.

That's it! You've had enough. Your boobs are aching, you still can't sit, you don't feel pretty, loved or sexually attractive. And now you have so much more to worry about, like if the baby is breathing, and whether or not you're a good mother. And due to your cracked nipples, you wonder if you're feeding your baby enough and if he'll die from malnutrition. You also wonder why all those moms in the breastfeeding books are smiling, and why you look like you have suffered infinite hours in a torture chamber as your little darling is suckling from your nipple. *What's wrong with me?* you might ask.

From my experience of dealing with many different patient types, I will say that the loony-tunes do best with the postpartum period. They tend to be more relaxed than they were prior to giving birth and downright doggone happy. The career-oriented neurotics are the worst because of the loss of control, and they expect too much from themselves. If you are in this category, just remember that you just went through a major ordeal. Give yourself a break, rest when you can, and try very hard to take care of yourself and your needs. Enlist the assistance of your friends and family, and spend quiet time with your partner.

FREQUENTLY ASKED QUESTIONS

When can I start exercising?

I firmly believe that exercise is a good thing to prevent postpartum depression. You shouldn't start too soon, however, because you will be quite wiped out. You should begin an exercise plan about 3 weeks after the birth if you've had a vaginal delivery, and 4 weeks after a C-section. Walking is a good thing to do early on in the exercise plan, and increase it gradually to an aerobic heart rate of 120 beats per minute, sustained for 15-20 minutes, at least 3 times per week. Gradually increase this to meet your exercise needs to help you lose weight, feel better and feel stronger. This also gives you time for yourself. It can be done when the baby naps or when you have a family member to sit with the baby.

Whatever you do, don't try to do too much too soon, as I have done. In my first pregnancy I was very discouraged about my postpartum weight, and having been on bed rest for preterm labor, I hadn't jogged or exercised for at least five months. I went to the track near my home and decided that I could at least run one mile. I was a marathon runner, after all. I was two weeks postpartum, and while I was running I began having chest pain and profuse sweating, and I became dizzy and light-headed. Of course, being the intelligent physician that I am, I didn't take any water with me for hydration. I rolled a little in the grass and dirt until I was able to lift myself to a nearby park bench. We didn't have cell phones then, so I waited, taking in my surroundings, until I found a mother of two and begged her to take me home. I was very fortunate that she did so despite my disheveled, frazzled, crazed, dirty and homeless appearance. The bottom line is, never do too much too soon.

When can I drive?

I prefer my patients not drive for 2-3 weeks after they deliver. As far as C-sections, I ask them to wait 4 weeks, because if they were involved in an accident it could put undue strain on the incision and perhaps cause tearing and herniation.

When can I have sex?

Most women don't ask this question unless they're under the age of 18, or unless they come to the postpartum visit with their partner. Most women do not feel like having sex for at least six weeks postpartum. When you go for your checkup, your physician will check you and see if your episiotomy site is well healed, or if your C-section scar is healed. Sex will be difficult at first, especially if you are breastfeeding. It affects the hormones, making the natural vaginal lubricant somewhat scant. There are plenty of over-the-counter remedies for this condition that you may wish to discuss with your health care provider.

When will I stop bleeding?

The answer to this varies for everyone; however, most of the time bleeding may occur on and off for a three-week interim. Near the end of the three weeks, it becomes a brownish spotting. Your next period may occur approximately 4-5 weeks later if you are not breastfeeding. Your first period may be heavy and last a little longer than it had in the past. If you go home and pass a large number of clots, and the bleeding doesn't lessen but remains heavier than a period, you should notify your practitioner. Delayed postpartum hemorrhages can occur, and your doctor should be made aware of any abnormal bleeding. Lochia, or the bleeding after delivery, has a different smell than normal menstrual blood. Don't be alarmed by this; it is normal.

When will I actually feel "in the mood" to have sex?

Remember, you have been through a huge physical and emotional change. Becoming a new mother has put quite a bit of strain on you both physically and emotionally. Allow your mind and body to heal simultaneously. Everyone is different, but don't expect too much too soon.

When will my vagina feel the way it used to?

I was amazed after I gave birth that it took at least four months to feel something reminiscent to what I felt prior to delivery. It can take a long time for the vagina to gain back its elasticity. The healing process at the site of the episiotomy is complete in 90 days. Therefore, if things feel strange, accept it and deal with it for at least 4 months. You'll be happier if you do so.

NINE MONTHS TO GO

My husband's penis keeps falling out of my vagina when we make love. Will it ever stay in there again?

Yes, as I mentioned before, as the vaginal mucosa gains back its elasticity, it also becomes tighter. Have no fear, your husband will not feel like Minnie Mouse forever. Your vagina will again contract as it did in the past.

I hate breastfeeding. Am I a horrible mother?

You're definitely not horrible, and if you even attempted it I think you're wonderful for doing so. Breastfeeding is not easy. It's time consuming, and if you're anything like me and can't sit still, it's quite difficult. It takes longer than bottle feeding and takes a lot more out of you physically. It does, however, burn quite a bit of calories and will aid in rapid weight loss, but it takes a lot of discipline on your part. You will have to maintain a healthy diet, and you will have more time restraints. And it's quite difficult to get any help from your partner on the feeding schedule, which is why I chose not to do it the second time as my life became more hectic. I do not feel that I neglected my second child while allowing my first to reap the benefits of suckling my bosom. As a matter of fact, after looking at me you might agree that my first child may actually be the one who was neglected.

Although breastfed infants can benefit from passive immunity the first three weeks of feeding, formula these days contains above and beyond the necessary nutritional requirements. Various formulas are more than adequate for a baby's growth and development. So keep that in mind, and by all means don't be guilt ridden if you choose to no longer breastfeed your infant. Remember that if you are nervous and agitated about feeding, and can't get the emotional and instructional support you need to do it effortlessly and adequately, you and your baby are better off not experiencing the turmoil.

What am I going to use for birth control?

That depends on when and if you wish to have another child. Keep in mind that you can get pregnant while nursing. Therefore, before you discuss the available options with your practitioner, make sure your partner uses a condom. You cannot take the standard birth control pill while breastfeeding because it diminishes breast milk. However, Depo-Provera, which is a progesterone-only medication given by injection, can be given four times a year and doesn't diminish the breast milk, and although it minimally crosses into the breast milk, it has no effects on the child. There are also progesterone-only birth control pills if you do not choose to take the shot.

Other options include an IUD, which should not be inserted until the uterus is back to its original size, usually 3 months postpartum. The same is true for a diaphragm, which should be inserted once the weight loss is within 10 pounds of your goal weight, since the vaginal size changes in conjunction with the amount of weight that one gains or loses. These options should be discussed at your postpartum visit. Sex should be avoided until you are comfortable with your birth control options. If you find it difficult to keep your partner away, it can't hurt to purchase an Uzi to keep in your nightstand table.

Are my nipples going to be black forever?

No, actually they are dark initially and probably up to three months after you deliver, until the melatonin (pigment hormone) decreases along with the other hormones of pregnancy.

Every time I breastfeed, my vagina "farts." Is this normal?

You must wonder if the great artists ever noticed this dilemma as they painted the varying Madonnas with Child. Certainly in the facial expressions in the works by Peter Paul Rubens and Leonardo DaVinci, one cannot imagine that they were privy to these nuances. Until the vagina gains back its elasticity, it tends to be lax. It, too, may contract, as does the uterus, with the stimulus of breastfeeding.

Passing gas is a common and natural event, and you should not worry; it will be short-lived. If you had a forceps delivery or a C-section and it continues beyond that point, you should make your practitioner aware.

My bladder is lazy and I keep wetting my pants. How long will this go on?

This can occur up to three months after you deliver. Give your body a chance, do Kegel exercises, and keep repeating to yourself that you have undergone a great experience and have a great gift, and now you need a big vacation.

How do I know if I am depressed?

If you find yourself not taking showers, locking your husband out of the house, not sleeping at night, or not having a desire to go anywhere or do anything, these could be signs of depression. You also may not want to care for your baby and may even resent him. Oftentimes family members, friends and your partner will recognize depression in you before you recognize it in yourself. I knew I was depressed when I didn't feel like shopping, and I had many opportunities to do so since my mother and mother-in-law were always readily available to babysit.

If you're prone to depression or have a history of depression in your family, you may wish to make your practitioner aware. Don't feel that you're abnormal. Too many new moms are embarrassed to express themselves because they feel that they should be on a high, but aren't. *Postpartum depression is a real and true entity.* If you think you are down, or have had a history of depression in the past, please, please, please call your practitioner. The sooner it is treated, the better for you and your baby. Treatments are safe, but may take a while to work, so they must be combined with psychotherapy.

Please give yourself a break and be proud of yourself—you've accomplished a lot. Just coming to the end of this book makes you an extra-special and unique individual. Be well, be happy and God bless you!

Index

A

Abdomen
    Pain, 42, 91, 100
    Stretch marks, 40, 75-76
Abortion
    Diagnosis of missed, 62, 100-101
    Previous pregnancy, 41, 57, 124
Abruptio placenta
    Signs of, 149
Accidents
    Types of injuries, 112
Acne, 94
Active (second) phase of labor, 167-185
Acupressure, 170
Acupuncture, 35, 96, 170, 175
Aerobics ,187
AFP (alpha fetal protein) screening, 67-68, 70, 87
    Triple screening, 67, 103
Age
    Amniocentesis, 60, 68-69, 82, 85-86
    Gestational ,31, 37, 55, 85-86, 121, 132, 139, 151, 158
Maternal, 43, 60-61, 68-70, 81-82, 133-135
Prenatal testing, 43, 60-61, 67-70, 81-84
Alcohol in pregnancy, 30, 56, 121, 151
Amniocentesis, xi, 60, 68-69, 82, 85-86, 123, 125
Amniotic fluid, 98, 112, 133, 141, 181
Analgesics, 72-73, 81, 97, 139, 169
Anemia, 59, 63, 65, 77
Anesthesia, 131, 168-170, 174, 176
Antacids, 33, 39
Anxiety, xiv, 22, 24, 28, 53, 87, 89, 91-92, 106, 116, 131-132, 137, 158, 169, 172, *see also* Worry
Aspartame, 30
Aspirin, 43, 73

B

Baby, *see also* Newborn
    Bonding with 184
    Conceiving, 22-23, 35-36
Back
    Exercise to strengthen, 78
    Pain, 29, 78, 106, 129-130, 153
Bath (hot tub), 81
Beta carotene, 31
Bicycling, 79
Biophysical profile, 132-135
Birth control, 24, 45-46, 189-190
Birth defects, 69, 80-88
Birth of baby
    Stages in, 158, 162, 165, 167, 173, 178
Birthing classes, 116-117
Bladder, 66, 78, 92, 106, 127, 144, 178-179, 190
Bleeding
    In early pregnancy, 41-42, 63, 73, 100-101
    In mid pregnancy, 124
    In late pregnancy, 148-150
Blood
    Banking your own, 146
    Bloody show, 160
    Clots, 97, 146, 188
    Concerns about transfusion, 146
    Pressure, 32, 36, 53, 55, 57, 64, 77, 102, 108, 133, 151, 170, 174
    Type, 63
Blood sugar, 56, 64, 77, 128, 133-134
Bowel movements, 33, 39, 97, 118, 131, 178, 182
Bras, 52, 103-104, 111, 118
Breast change, 34, 38, 50, 75, 89, 93, 95, 127
Breast milk, 75, 118, 127, 189-190
Breastfeeding, 186-190
Breath, shortness of, 127, 138, 151
Breech, xv-xvii, 42, 141-142, 145, 147, 177

C

Calcium, 26, 30-31, 39, 99, 113-114, 121, 151
Calories, 30-33, 35, 72, 77, 96, 102, 189
Carbohydrates, 30, 33-34
Carpal tunnel syndrome, 111, 115
Cats, 64-65
Cephalopelvic disproportion, 147, 176
Cervix,
    Changes in, 135, 152, 163, 169
    Dilation, 137, 149-151, 158, 160
    Effacement, 73, 137, 149-151, 158, 160
    Incompetence, 43, 57, 77, 123, 153
Caesarian section
    Emergency, 124, 142, 169, 174, 176-177
    Exercise following, 186-187
    Fear of, 143
    Vaginal birth after (VBAC), 15, 146-147
Chicken pox, 47
Childbirth
    Concerns about, 15-16, 142, 148
    Education, 116-117, 178
Chlamydia, *see* Sexually transmitted diseases
Cigarettes, 110, 112, *see also* Smoking; Tobacco
Clothing, 97, 107, 110, 140
Colostrum, 130
Conception, *see* Baby, conceiving
Constipation, xii, 31-32, 39, 92, 98, 108, 117-118, 127, 129
Contractions
    Braxton-Hicks, 108, 130
    False labor, 157
    First stage of labor, 149, 158, 162
    Premature, 73, 75, 118, 151-153
    Second phase of labor, 171, 173, 182
Cravings, *see* Food
Chorionic villus sampling, 60, 68-69, 83-86, 103

D

Delivery, positions for, 180-182; *see also* Childbirth
Delivery room, 181
Demerol, 169, 172
Depression, 71, 185-186, 191
DES daughters, 46, 100
Diabetes, gestational, 29, 36, 56, 58, 64, 102, 125, 128, 134, 139, 145, 177
Diarrhea, 99, 158
Diet, 29-35, 41, 56, 58, 71, 99, 119, 134, 139, 189
Dilation, 56, 73, 77, 85, 137, 149-151, 153, 158, 164, 169, 171, 178
Doctor, choosing, 1-8, 12-19; *see also* Physician; Obstetrician
Down syndrome, 60, 66-70, 82-83, 87-88
Drugs
    Recreational, 30, 56, 112, 151
    Therapeutic, *see* Medication
Due date, xvii, 23, 27, 48-49, 56, 136, 150, 154

E

Eating, 24-36, 64-65, 71-72, 98-99, 119-121
Eclampsia, 57, 133-135, 145
Ectopic, 42, 44, 46, 62, 100
Edema (swelling), 32, 76, 80, 102, 111, 113-114, 125, 129-130, 133-134, 145, 184
Effacement, 73, 137, 149-151, 158, 164
Emotions in pregnancy, 12, 74-75, 91, 130, 159, 188-189
Endometriosis, 45
Energy, 103, 159
Engagement of fetus in pelvis, 142
Epidural, 131-132, 169-174, 176
Episiotomy, 80, 174, 184, 187-189
Estimated date of delivery, 24, 48
Exercise
    in pregnancy, 11, 29, 56, 76-79, 114
    postpartum, 186-187

F

False labor, *See* Labor, false
Fatty acids, xi, 25-28, 119
Family history, 22, 58, 64, 84, 152, 134, 191
Fatigue, 39, 72, 91,
Fetal
    activity, 113, 129, 133
    development, 25, 31, 81, 86-87, 99-100, 106, 119, 121-122, 133
    distress, 57, 135, 145, 147, 155, 169, 174, 176
    heartbeat, 37, 53, 89, 96, 109, 132, 155, 163
    lung maturity, 48, 124, 135, 152
    monitoring, 145, 151, 155, 163, 167, 176,
    movement, 85, 113, 122, 129
Fibroids, 42-43, 58, 62, 151
First trimester screening, 63, 67-69, 82-84, 103
    Sequential screening, 43, 60, 62, 65, 68-70, 84, 103
Fluids, 34, 72, 92, 97, 121, 148
Folic acid, 25-26
Food
    Aversions, 108
    Cravings, 108, 120
Forceps, 6, 15, 57, 131, 145, 169, 173-174, 190

G

Gas
    Foods that produce, 93
    Intestinal, 93, 190
Glucola, 56, 128, 134
Gonorrhea, *see* Sexually transmitted diseases

H

Hemorrhoids, x-xi, 39, 77, 108, 117, 127, 154, 178
Herpes, 44-45, 147-148
Home pregnancy test, 36-37, 51

Hospital
    Concerns about, 2, 162-163
    Getting to, 162
Hot tubs, 81
Hyperemesis, 34, 101
Hypertension, 29, 58, 145,
Hypnotist, 131-132, 170, 174

I

Illness in pregnancy, 36, 63, 65, 80-81, 133
Immunization, 47, 125
Incompetent cervix, *See* cervix
Indigestion, 39, 98, 129, 158
Induction of labor, 48, 56, 73, 85, 135-137, 150
Infection, 32, 44-45, 47, 55, 58, 61-66, 79, 120, 123, 133, 135,
    151-153, 161-162, 181
Intercourse, 73-74, 76, 124, 148
Internal fetal monitoring, *see* Fetal, monitoring
Intrauterine growth restriction (IUGR), 133

J

Job
    Lifting during pregnancy, 106

K

Kegel, 76, 118, 144, 182, 190

L

Labia, 74, 76, 80, 184
Labor
    Duration, 158, 161, 169, 176
    False, 157, 161-162
    First phase, 158, 165
    Induction of, 48, 73, 85, 135-136

Preterm, 10, 32, 47, 73, 75, 77, 102, 105, 118, 120, 123, 145, 150-154
  Second phase, 167, 173, 176, 178-184
  Signs of, 149-150, 153, 159-162
Labor and delivery rooms, 2, 181
Labor pain, relief of, 6, 116-117, 131, 137-138, 168-176
Lactation, *see* Breast milk; Breastfeeding
Lanugo, 183
Latent phase, *see* Labor, first phase
Leg cramps, 97, 108, 113-114
Leukorrhea, 179
Ligament pain, 42, 108, 111
Lochia, 188
Lovemaking, 73-75, 189-190
Lyme disease, 65

M

Macrosomia, 139, 141-142
Magnesium sulfate, 10, 151
Making love, *see* Lovemaking
Mask of pregnancy, 41
Massage in labor, 175, 184
Maternal age, *see* Age
Maternal serum alpha-fetal protein screening, *see* AFP
Maternity clothes, *see* Clothing
Measles, 47
Medication, 3, 10, 24, 34-36, 39, 41, 44-47, 59, 72-73, 80-81, 94, 123, 145, 151, 162, 169-173, 176
Membranes
  Premature rupture of, 123
  Rupture of, 154, 161
Menstrual period, 23, 36-37, 49, 100-101, 190
Midwife, xv, 1, 12, 14-15
Milk (drinking), 30-31, 64, 87, 96, 99, 113, 120
Miscarriage
  Diagnosis, 46, 100-101
  Risk of, 44, 46, 63, 120

Morning sickness, 34, 91, 95
Mucous plug, 160
Multiple gestation, 31, *see also* Twins

N

Narcotics, 158, 165, 168, 172, 180
Nasal congestion, 125, 127
Nausea, 25, 30, 33-35, 38, 41, 52, 91, 98, 100-102
Neural tube defects, 25, 67, 87, 98
Newborn, 61-62, 181,183-184, 187, 193
Nipples, 38, 40, 50, 75, 93, 118, 155, 184, 186, 190
Non-stress test (NST), 132, 134
Nosebleeds, 9
Nutrasweet, *see* Aspartame
Nutrition in pregnancy, 72, 76, 101, *see also* Diet

O

Obese, 28, 139
Obstetrician, x, 1, 5-8, 13-19, 36-38, 41, 43-44, 48, 55, 86, 117,
    see also Doctor; Physician
Odors, 79, 94,
Oligohydramnious, 125
Oral sex, 94
Orgasm, 73-74, 80, 150

P

Pain, 38, 41-43, 45, 85, 91, 100-101, 114, 129-130, 138-139,
    141, 153, 162
    relief of, *see* Labor pain, relief of; Medication; Tylenol
Pap smear, 57-58, 61-62
Physical activity, 91, *see also* Exercise
Physician, choosing, 1-8, 12-19, *see also* Obstetrician; Doctor
Pigmentation, 38, 40-41, 190
Pitocin, xvii, 170-171, 173
Placenta previa, 73, 77, 124, 142, 148-149
Polyhydramnious, 124-125, 133

Position
    For delivery, 180, 182
    Of baby, 68, 122, 141, 176-177, 183, *see also* Breech
Postpartum bleeding, xvi, 188
Practitioner, *see* Midwife; Obstetrician; Physician
Pre-eclampsia, 57, 133-135, 145, *see also* Blood, pressure;
        Pregnancy, hypertension induced by; Toxemia
Pregnancy
    Hypertension, induced by, 29, 32, 37, 58, 64, 77, 102, 133,
        145, *see also* Blood, pressure; Pre-eclampsia
    Loss of, 43, 84, *see also* Miscarriage
    Test, 36-37, 51-52
Premature labor (preterm labor), *see* Labor, preterm
Premilk (colostrum), 130
Prostaglandins to ripen cervix, 73, 154
Protein (in diet), 30-31, 35, 99, 119

R

Regional nerve block, 173
Relaxation, exercises for, 116-117, 172
Rh factor, 63, 125

S

Saliva, 92-93
Salt, 32
Saunas, 81
Sequential screening, xi, 43, 60, 62, 65, 68-70, 84, 103
Sexual relations, *see* Lovemaking
Sexually transmitted diseases (STDs), 44, 58, 61-63, 78, 85
Shortness of breath, *see* Breath, shortness of
Shoulder dystocia, 29, 177
Sitz baths, 118
Skiing, 79
Sleep, 34, 40, 77, 89, 91, 96-97, 103, 111, 114, 117-118, 127, 130, 191
Smoking, 36, 56, 98, 110, 112, 133-134, 151, *see also* Cigarettes;
        Tobacco

Snacks, 30-31, 35, 96
Spinal block, *see* Epidural
Strep, Group B, 55, 58, 135, 150, 161
Stretch marks, *see* Abdomen, stretch marks
Syphilis, *see* Sexually transmitted diseases

T

Teeth, 47-48
Tennis, 79, 94
TENS, 175
Tobacco, 30, *see also* Cigarettes; Smoking
Toxemia, 32, 77, 133, *see also* Pre-eclampsia
Twins, xv-xvi, 24, 31, 62, 77, 102, 144-145
Tylenol, 72-73, 81, 97, 139

U

Ultrasound, 37, 42, 46, 53, 55, 60-63, 66-68, 70, 82-83, 85-87, 102, 103, 122, 124, 133, 145, 148, 152-153, 177
Umbilical cord
    Nuchal cord, 183
    Prolapse of, 142
Undergarments, 110-111, *see also* Bras
Urinary incontinence, 127, 130, 143-144, 190
Urinary tract infection, 32, 58, 65-66
Urination, 34, 66, 76-77, 92, 106
Urine sample/specimen, 52, 55, 65, 108, 133
Uterine incision, 146, 187
Uterus, 39, 42, 58, 60, 62, 78-79, 85, 91-92, 94, 96, 100, 102, 108, 117, 123-124, 132, 138, 141, 145-146, 148, 151-153, 155, 158, 162, 170-171, 184, 190

V

Vagina, 62, 66, 73, 76, 148-150, 152, 174, 178-182, 184, 186-188, 190
    Discharge, 79, 94, 100, 149, 160
    Infection, 55, 79, 110
Vaginal delivery, 15, 29, 71, 110, 136, 145-148, 177, 181, 186

Varicose veins (varicosities), x, 29, 48, 71, 93, 97, 102, 108, 114, 130
VBAC (vaginal birth after c-section), 146-147
Vegetables and fruit, 30-31, 65, 93, 99, 111
Vitamins, 3, 24-26, 30-31, 33, 35, 37, 39, 75, 91, 98-99, 102, 111, 114, 117, 118, 148, 185

W

Walking, 91, 154, 187
    During labor, 10, 131, 162, 164, 176
Water, breaking of, *see* Membranes
Weight gain, 28-31, 40, 70-72, 75-76, 95-97, 102, 125, 133-134, 139, 151, 177
Wine, *see* Alcohol
Work, 39-40, 56, 63, 65, 105-107
Worry, xiv-xv, 11, 21, 24, 27, 89, 102, 125, 131, 140, 161, 181, 186, *see also* Anxiety

Y

Yoga, 96, 170, 174
Yogurt, 30-31, 99